Coping After COVID-19

Coping After COVID-19

Cognitive Behavioral Skills for Anxiety, Depression, and Adjusting to Chronic Illness

THERAPIST GUIDE

ABHISHEK JAYWANT

LAUREN E. OBERLIN

STEPHANIE CHERESTAL

CHRISTINA BUENO CASTELLANO

VICTORIA M. WILKINS

DORA KANELLOPOULOS

OXFORD
UNIVERSITY PRESS

OXFORD
UNIVERSITY PRESS

Oxford University Press is a department of the University of Oxford. It furthers
the University's objective of excellence in research, scholarship, and education
by publishing worldwide. Oxford is a registered trade mark of Oxford University
Press in the UK and certain other countries.

Published in the United States of America by Oxford University Press
198 Madison Avenue, New York, NY 10016, United States of America.

Library of Congress Cataloging-in-Publication Data
Names: Jaywant, Abhishek, author.
Title: Coping after COVID-19 : cognitive behavioral skills for anxiety,
depression, and adjusting to chronic illness - therapist guide /
Abhishek Jaywant, Lauren E. Oberlin, Stephanie Cherestal,
Christina Bueno-Castellano, Victoria M. Wilkins, Dora Kanellopoulos.
Description: New York, NY : Oxford University Press, [2024] |
Includes bibliographical references and index. |
Identifiers: LCCN 2023019553 (print) | LCCN 2023019554 (ebook) |
ISBN 9780197699379 (paperback) | ISBN 9780197699393 (epub) |
ISBN 9780197699409
Subjects: LCSH: COVID-19 (Disease)—Complications. |
COVID-19 (Disease)—Patients—Rehabilitation.
Classification: LCC RA644.C67 J393 2023 (print) | LCC RA644.C67 (ebook) |
DDC 616.2/4144—dc23/eng/20230710
LC record available at https://lccn.loc.gov/2023019553
LC ebook record available at https://lccn.loc.gov/2023019554

DOI: 10.1093/med-psych/9780197699379.001.0001

Printed by Marquis Book Printing, Canada

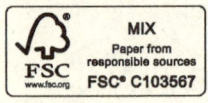

Stunning developments in healthcare have taken place over the last several years, but many of our widely accepted interventions and strategies in mental health and behavioral medicine have been brought into question by research evidence as not only lacking benefit but perhaps inducing harm (Barlow, 2010). Other strategies have been proven effective using the best current standards of evidence, resulting in broad-based recommendations to make these practices more available to the public (McHugh & Barlow, 2010). Several recent developments are behind this revolution. First, we have arrived at a much deeper understanding of pathology, both psychological and physical, which has led to the development of new, more precisely targeted interventions. Second, our research methodologies have improved substantially, such that we have reduced threats to internal and external validity, making the outcomes more directly applicable to clinical situations. Third, governments around the world and healthcare systems and policymakers have decided that the quality of care should improve, that it should be evidence-based, and that it is in the public's interest to ensure that this happens (Barlow, 2004; Institute of Medicine, 2001, 2015; McHugh & Barlow, 2010).

Of course, the major stumbling block for clinicians everywhere is the accessibility of newly developed evidence-based psychological interventions. Workshops and books can go only so far in acquainting responsible and conscientious practitioners with the latest behavioral healthcare practices and their applicability to individual patients. This series, Treatments *ThatWork*™, is devoted to communicating these exciting new interventions to clinicians on the frontlines of practice.

The manuals and workbooks in this series contain step-by-step detailed procedures for assessing and treating specific problems and diagnoses.

But this series also goes beyond the books and manuals by providing ancillary materials that will approximate the supervisory process in assisting practitioners in the implementation of these procedures in their practice.

In our emerging healthcare system, the growing consensus is that evidence-based practice offers the most responsible course of action for the mental health professional. All behavioral healthcare clinicians deeply desire to provide the best possible care for their patients. In this series, our aim is to close the dissemination and information gap and make that possible.

This Therapist Guide is designed for individuals experiencing persistent symptoms of COVID-19 and co-occurring anxiety, depression, or difficulty adjusting to the illness. This post infection condition is often referred to as long COVID. It is now well recognized that some individuals who contract COVID-19 will experience lingering symptoms such as fatigue, changes in movement and sensation, cognitive difficulties, and shortness of breath, among other health challenges. The authors draw on their experience working with individuals with COVID-19 starting in 2020 on the frontlines of the pandemic. The treatment program is based on a cognitive behavioral model that describes how unhelpful thoughts, distressing emotions, and maladaptive avoidance behaviors interact with persisting symptoms of COVID-19 to perpetuate distress and disability.

The Therapist Guide contains many useful skills that target these thoughts, emotions, and behaviors with the goal of alleviating anxiety and depression and bolstering coping skills for managing medical symptoms. Also included are strategies to manage cognitive difficulties and fatigue, techniques for addressing loss and grief, and adaptations when working with individuals from culturally diverse backgrounds. The techniques and skills described here will be an important resource for clinicians working with clients who struggle with persistent symptoms of COVID-19.

David H. Barlow, Editor-in-Chief
Treatments *ThatWork*™
Boston, Massachusetts

References

Barlow, D. H. (2004). Psychological treatments. *American Psychologist, 59*, 869–878.

Barlow, D. H. (2010). Negative effects from psychological treatments: A perspective. *American Psychologist, 65*(2), 13–20.

Institute of Medicine. (2001). *Crossing the quality chasm: A new health system for the 21st century.* National Academy Press.

Institute of Medicine. (2015). *Psychosocial interventions for mental and substance use disorders: A framework for establishing evidence-based standards.* National Academies Press.

McHugh, R. K., & Barlow, D. H. (2010). Dissemination and implementation of evidence-based psychological interventions: A review of current efforts. *American Psychologist, 65*(2), 73–84.

Contents

PART II: ADDITIONAL CLINICAL APPLICATIONS

Introduction and Setting the Stage

COVID-19 has exacted a devastating global toll. Vaccines and antiviral treatments have had a significant effect in mitigating serious illness and death, but despite medical and pharmacological advances in prevention and treatment, new infections continue to occur as of the time of writing. Some individuals who contract COVID-19 experience persistent symptoms of the illness, even after the acute infection. These symptoms tend to be more common in individuals who were hospitalized, but persisting symptoms can also occur in those with a mild initial infection. Anxiety, depression, cognitive symptoms, and fatigue are common sequelae of COVID-19 (Vanderlind et al., 2021).

Drawing on our experience treating the emotional and psychological sequelae of other medical illnesses, we developed a treatment program to address anxiety and depression in survivors of COVID-19. The program was developed and implemented rapidly during the initial waves of the COVID-19 pandemic in New York City. We drew heavily from cognitive behavioral therapy (CBT), acceptance and commitment therapy (ACT), existing psychotherapy approaches for individuals with medical illnesses (Alexopoulos et al., 2012, 2018), and mindfulness-based strategies in a culturally informed manner. Our approach was iteratively refined as we listened to and learned from the challenges that clients with COVID-19 faced. We first implemented interventions described in this treatment program on inpatient medical rehabilitation units in individual and group sessions. We found that among clients with COVID-19 on these inpatient units who engaged in our treatment program, 67 percent did not need follow-up psychiatric care on discharge (Jaywant et al., 2021).

We concurrently developed a parallel outpatient program for clients recently discharged from the hospital. Interventions were implemented in weekly individual and group formats. Working with clients in the community gave us additional opportunities to learn from the experience of COVID-19 survivors and iterate, refine, and adapt our approach. We analyzed depression and anxiety severity scores at treatment initiation and discharge from this outpatient program and found improvements in both (Park et al., 2023). Two additional randomized controlled trials—with overlapping components with our approach—have provided support for cognitive behavioral interventions in treating anxiety and depression after COVID-19 (Li et al., 2020; Liu et al., 2021).

Is This Treatment Program Right for You and Your Client?

This treatment program is designed for individuals recovering from COVID-19 who experience residual and persistent medical/physical symptoms of COVID-19 with co-occurring anxiety, depression, and difficulty adjusting to the illness. We also include modules designed to help clients manage COVID-19-related cognitive symptoms, fatigue, and sleep disturbance. The treatment program is not intended to "cure" or directly treat the medical/physical symptoms of COVID-19 themselves, which typically requires interdisciplinary medical care and rehabilitation. However, it can be an important ingredient of helping your client adjust to illness and improve functioning. In a retrospective analysis of 106 individuals hospitalized for COVID-19 who were undergoing inpatient physical rehabilitation, we compared 43 individuals who were referred to and completed at least one session of our CBT program to 63 individuals who did not participate in our CBT program (Patel et al., 2021). Compared to those individuals who did not engage in our program, those who did had greater gains in physical function and self-care skills.

This Therapist Guide contains familiar content and techniques for therapists trained in CBT and related modalities. Those who practice other modalities of psychotherapy will also find the content and techniques to be helpful, particularly as our experience suggests that many individuals recovering from COVID-19 desire concrete skills to better manage their symptoms. Our program has not been designed for, nor evaluated in, clients with primary diagnoses of post-traumatic stress disorder (PTSD), alcohol/substance use disorder, or psychosis.

Therapist Note

Many terms have been used to describe the phenomenon of persisting COVID-19 symptoms. The community of survivors, particularly those who suffered only mild initial infections but have persisting symptoms, tend to favor use of the term "long COVID" or "long-haul COVID." The National Institutes of Health has adopted the term "post-acute sequelae of COVID-19" (PASC) in its research initiatives and funding. Those who were hospitalized with severe illness requiring intensive care are also sometimes classified as having "post-intensive care syndrome" (PICS). In this Therapist Guide, we use terminology that is descriptive and broad, such as "persisting symptoms of COVID-19," to remain inclusive of all the above terms. However, if your client has a preferred term, then it may be most helpful to use their language and terminology.

Therapist Note

Research on COVID-19 is rapidly evolving, and the tools and techniques in this program should not be considered definitive or all-encompassing. We recommend you review recent research literature when working with clients with persisting symptoms of COVID-19. We strongly recommend that you adopt a curious, open, and flexible stance to your client's symptom presentation, goals, and techniques used, especially as COVID-19 is a remarkably heterogenous condition.

How to Use This Book and Implement This Treatment Program

This treatment program is intended to be implemented in a modular, flexible manner. Each module will often require more than one session. Within each module (chapter), we provide a suggested number of sessions. Some clients may benefit from progressing through the modules (chapters) as presented, while for others, the order in which you implement modules will depend on your client's presenting concerns and goals and your conceptualization of the primary targets of treatment. Figure I.1 is a *suggested* order of modules depending on client presentation and case conceptualization. We recommend that all therapists read and

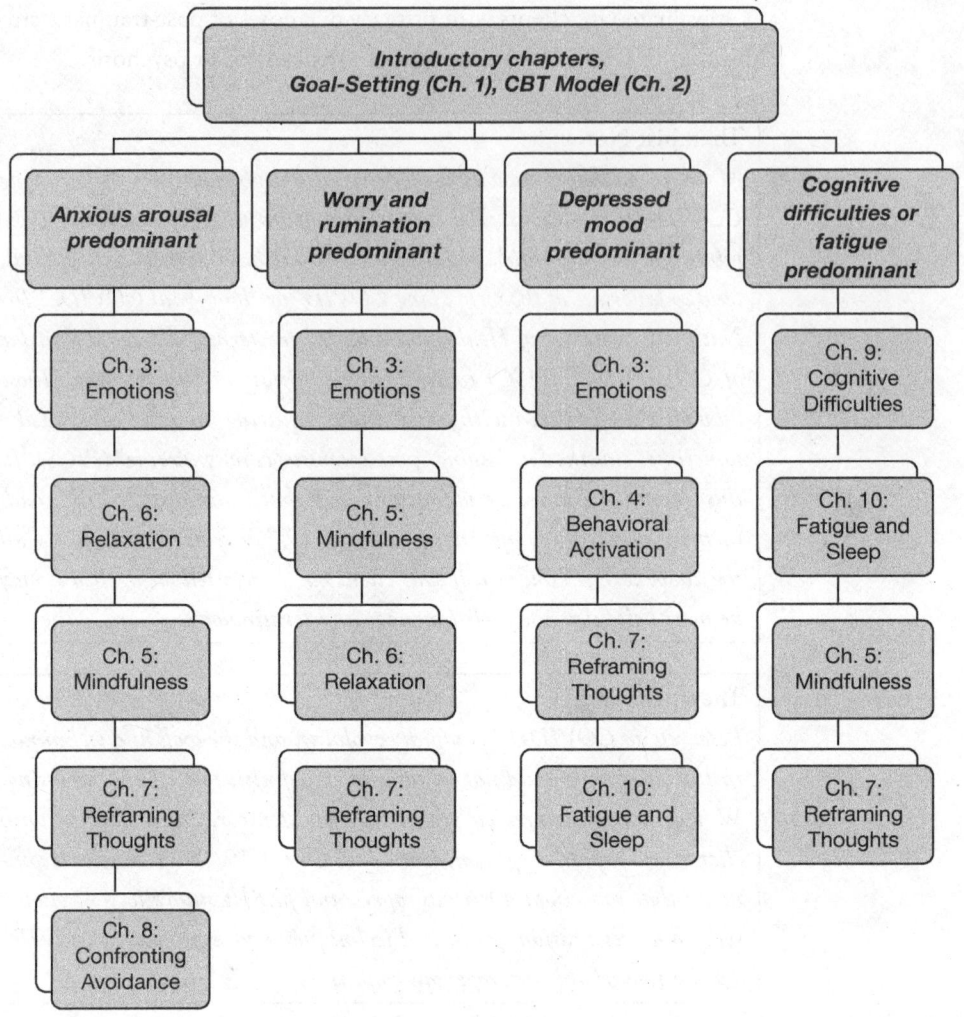

Figure I.1.

Suggested Sequence of Modules/Chapters Based on Predominant Symptom Target. These are recommended based on the authors' experience and should be tailored to the individual client. Most clients will benefit from Chapter 11 (Participating in Medical Treatment) and Chapter 12 (Putting It All Together and Managing Uncertainty).

familiarize themselves with the content in this introduction. Some clients may also benefit from the additional clinical applications in Chapters 13 and 14 (Loss and Grief; Caregivers and Families). To facilitate treatment, we recommend that your client purchase the accompanying Client

Workbook. Worksheets are available in both the Therapist Guide and Client Workbook or can be accessed by searching for this book's title on the Oxford Academic platform, at academic.oup.com.

Considerations When Working with Clients Experiencing Persisting Symptoms of COVID-19

Staying Up to Date on Treatment Information

With new variants, treatments, ebbs and flows of infection risk, and evolving public health guidelines, we recommend that you stay as up to date as possible on the information most relevant to your client. At the minimum, familiarity with current guidelines from the U.S. Centers for Disease Control and Prevention (CDC) or other relevant public health body can help you to conceptualize whether your client's thoughts and behaviors are accurate or whether they contain cognitive distortions and maladaptive avoidance.

Invisible Symptoms and Stigma

Like many individuals who live with chronic medical and mental illnesses, individuals with persistent symptoms of COVID-19 often feel as if they suffer with an invisible illness. Others may not recognize the internal distress or difficulty your client has, which creates a mismatch between others' expectations and your client's abilities. On the other end, clients left with visible aftereffects of COVID-19 (e.g., those who require supplemental oxygen, or who walk with a cane or other assistive device) may experience stigma. Stigma can lead others to avoid the client, treat them differently, or convey the message that the client is somehow to blame or at fault for what they are experiencing. If these themes come up in your work with your client, we recommend acknowledging and validating this experience, and using the tools in this Therapist Guide as well as your therapeutic skills to help the client communicate their experience to others in their life in a way that is genuine and authentic to them.

Resilience and Gratitude

Individuals with persisting symptoms of COVID-19 can be remarkably resilient. We have worked with medically hospitalized clients who, after spending weeks on ventilators, motivated themselves day after day to persist in their rehabilitation and expressed a profound gratitude for a chance to reaffirm their commitment to the people and experiences in their life who matter the most. Clients find small ways to adapt, to find meaning, and to grow. We have found it helpful when implementing this treatment program to keep clients' innate resilience in mind and to know that part of your role is to use the skills and strategies in this program to bolster clients' own resilience and coping tools. Validation and positive reinforcement of strengths should be a part of your work with your client. If your client expresses gratitude at new perspectives gained, we recommend highlighting the perspectives gained and reinforcing positive affect and gratitude.

The Disproportionate Impact on Clients from Diverse Socioeconomic, Linguistic, and Ethnic Backgrounds

The COVID-19 pandemic highlighted many existing structural and systemic inequities in the United States healthcare system, which may also be present in other countries. In the early wave of the pandemic in the United States, Black and Hispanic Americans suffered the effects of COVID-19 disproportionately. Much of our experience developing this treatment program came from working with clients from underserved and disadvantaged backgrounds. Our cognitive behavioral model of COVID-19 includes a key role for environmental stressors such as racial injustice and financial instability in the adjustment difficulty your client may experience.

Key Treatment Ingredients

Psychoeducation

In this population, psychoeducation is a critical ingredient of treatment. Many individuals who experience persisting symptoms of COVID-19 have no history of mental illness, psychiatric care, or psychotherapy. Thus, increasing emotional awareness and discussing the interaction and bidirectional association between thoughts/emotions and physical/medical symptoms can be a significant paradigm shift for many who may have traditionally viewed the mind and body as separate. Describing how emotions such as fear, anxiety, sadness, and anger are normative in the context of severe medical illness can similarly be novel information for many clients. Educating your client on the most current research on COVID-19 is also important.

Acknowledging Physical Symptoms as Real, Distressing, and Debilitating

Many individuals recovering from COVID-19 who have persisting symptoms report feeling dismissed and ignored by their family, their friends, and even their medical providers. This is especially true for those with mild initial infections. Accumulating evidence supports the potential role of inflammatory, autoimmune, cardiovascular, or central nervous system mechanisms in the persistence of COVID-19 symptoms. It is therefore critical to validate and acknowledge your client's symptoms as "real"—in other words, COVID-19 symptoms are not just the psychosomatic manifestation of depression, anxiety, or other psychiatric illness. However, anxiety, depression, and emotional distress can perpetuate and exacerbate symptoms of COVID-19. Each client's emotional reaction to medical/physical illness is unique and valid, and each client needs empathy and can benefit from the skills in this program.

Building Agency in the Face of Loss of Autonomy and Independence

Like many medical illnesses, COVID-19 can affect a client's sense of autonomy and independence. Whereas prior to contracting COVID-19 a client may have been fully independent in their daily activities, they may now require assistance and support from others. Even clients with milder infections may experience symptoms that require help from others—as in the case of an individual with fatigue who needs their significant other to help with grocery shopping, meal preparation, or childcare. These experiences can lead to a feeling of lost autonomy and identity. Clients can struggle to come to terms with these changes, yearning for the independence they had prior to COVID-19. The skills and techniques learned in this program can give clients a greater sense of autonomy and control over their situation, which in turn can foster acceptance, resilience, and growth.

Interdisciplinary Collaboration

Individuals with persisting symptoms of COVID-19 typically present with a constellation of medical, physical, and emotional difficulties. Managing symptoms of COVID-19 requires an interdisciplinary approach where psychotherapy is one component of a larger care plan. We recommend working in close collaboration with your client's medical providers. Open dialogue—with the client's permission—can assist you in conceptualizing which of your client's thoughts and beliefs may be consistent with their current physical and medical limitations and which may be cognitive distortions.

Inclusion of Family Members and Caregivers

Family members and caregivers can be valuable allies and partners in your client's recovery journey. We recommend exploring with your client the possibility of having a family member, significant other, or caregiver participate in psychotherapy sessions when clinically indicated. Family members and caregivers can provide valuable insight into the client's daily function, support the client in homework completion, and help to mitigate barriers to implementing cognitive behavioral strategies.

Homework and Out-of-Session Practice

As in most traditional CBT programs, it is important to have your client practice skills out of session using worksheets and homework exercises. At-home practice exercises reinforce concepts learned in session, enable your client to incorporate skills into their daily life, and help you and your client to troubleshoot barriers and pitfalls. Repeated practice makes skill use more automatic and routine, enables clients to increase autonomy and self-efficacy, and is overall a key component of treatment success. We recommend that you explain the importance of at-home exercises upfront when initiating treatment. If you find that your client responds negatively to the term "homework," then it can be useful to refer instead to "at-home practice exercises" or "out-of-session practice." In each core module in this treatment program, we include descriptions of suggested homework exercises.

Additional Factors in Treatment Delivery

Telehealth

We found in implementing this program that many clients enjoyed the ease and convenience of telehealth-based psychotherapy. For others, significant challenges can emerge around internet connectivity, comfort with using technology, and lack of privacy at home. These challenges can be especially salient to individuals from diverse sociocultural and ethnic backgrounds where intergenerational living may be more common. When implementing this treatment program, we recommend weighing the costs and benefits of in-person versus telehealth implementation and problem-solving barriers to telehealth if that is the chosen modality. Solutions to privacy issues that we used included scheduling sessions while family members or housemates were working or in school; siting in the backyard or in a stationary car; or picking an enclosed but remote location in the home where household members are less likely to disturb the client.

Working with Clients Whose Views on the Pandemic Differ from Yours

Individuals who present to this treatment program may differ from each other and from you. They will likely have diverse cultural backgrounds, life experiences, values, and views on the world around them. Differences in beliefs surrounding the impact of the pandemic are common, as are beliefs on how one ought to continue to engage with the world around one. When working with clients in this treatment program, you may meet with clients whose views related to vaccines and infection mitigation strategies differ. In such situations, we encourage you to practice mindful awareness of your own views, the views of the client, and your responses to differences that arise. We encourage displaying empathy and respect for your client's views even if they might differ from your own, and work on increasing the client's motivation to follow the recommendations and advice of their medical providers. It can sometimes be helpful for you as the therapist to ask permission from your client to provide education that would be helpful to them, such as research surrounding the COVID-19 vaccines, and present any education in a straightforward manner without forcing any personal beliefs upon the client.

Collaborative Empiricism

The notion of collaborative empiricism and hypothesis-testing is a fundamental value underlying CBT approaches to treating psychological disorders. We find collaborative empiricism to be especially helpful when working with clients with persistent symptoms of COVID-19, a relatively new illness where new knowledge is rapidly evolving. We recommend that you maintain a curious mindset in which you and the client collaborate to uncover factors that perpetuate or exacerbate symptoms as well as factors that alleviate symptoms. This collaborative process is most effective when done in a manner that is nonjudgmental and empathic and reduces potential power differentials between you and the client. This approach is especially helpful when you as the therapist identify with a dominant cultural background and your client identifies with an underrepresented group.

Therapist Burnout

The COVID-19 pandemic has been unique in that therapists and healthcare providers globally have endured similar external stressors and uncertainty as clients and are likely to have been infected with COVID-19 themselves. Further, mental health providers of all disciplines are experiencing significant demand for their services. When implementing this treatment, it is important to attend to your own mental health and well-being, and to be aware of any of your own thoughts and emotions that may arise in response to discussing certain topics with your client (for example, related to beliefs around vaccination), particularly if you have experienced your own stress or loss associated with COVID-19.

> **Therapist Note**
> *Pharmacological treatment can be an important component of post-COVID-19 care, particularly in managing depression, anxiety, and cognitive symptoms. This treatment program can be implemented in concert with prescribed psychotropic medications.*

Application of This Program to Anxiety and Depression in Other Medical Conditions

Although this treatment program was developed for individuals with persistent symptoms of COVID-19, the tools and techniques here may be helpful for clients who experience a sudden and debilitating medical illness, with persistent residual symptoms, and co-occurring difficulty in emotional adjustment, anxiety, and depression.

Assessment and Symptom Tracking

Here we introduce approaches to an initial intake assessment and techniques for symptom monitoring. One intake session may be sufficient, although an initial assessment may need to be broken up into multiple sessions, particularly if your client experiences fatigue and/or has a complex medical and psychiatric history.

Preparing for the Intake

When scheduling the intake, provide the client with a brief overview of the intake assessment, and explain how information gathered during the intake is meant to guide treatment planning. Ask the client to provide a list of medications, relevant medical records, and a list of current providers.

Language and communication preferences should be elicited prior to the first session. It is important to ask about your client's comfort and proficiency when speaking, writing, and reading in English to determine their ability to comprehend the consent process, complete self-report measures, and understand concepts discussed in treatment. If a language barrier is identified, you should first determine if there are feasible alternative providers for the client to receive care in their native and/or preferred language. To help determine whether you should refer the client to another provider, consider whether there are other therapists who are (1) fluent in the client's preferred language; (2) competent in treating this client population; and (3) able to provide accessible treatment to the client.

Clients who have immigrated from another country may change their name or adopt an anglicized name to assimilate. Clients who no longer identify with birth names that misgendered them may prefer to be addressed by a different name as well. Discussing name and pronoun preferences at the onset of treatment is therefore an important consideration.

Because there were no feasible alternative providers when we developed this treatment program, we occasionally implemented this treatment program using an interpreter. If you use an interpreter, avoid using family or friends of the client, because doing so can create privacy concerns and introduce additional biases. Use a certified interpreter who is proficient in speaking, reading, and writing in English and in the client's preferred language. Interpreters familiar with the client's ethnocultural background may be better equipped to convey specific nonverbal mannerisms, cultural customs, slang, and expectations. Note that interpreters are not necessarily bound by the same confidentiality laws as mental health providers, and this information should be conveyed to the client prior to consenting to begin treatment. It may be reassuring to the client to have the interpreter sign a confidentiality agreement prior to treatment.

If you use an interpreter, meet with them prior to the intake. Explain that you would like them to interpret what you say, without omitting, adding, or altering the meaning of information being conveyed. Ask the interpreter to let you know if translations distort the original meaning of the message and/or technique being discussed in session. During the session, the interpreter should sit beside the client and interpret information verbatim, in the first person. While engaging in the session, you should face the client and speak directly to them, and not the interpreter. Use hand gestures and/or body language as you would use to convey empathy and compassion to English-speaking clients in session. While in session with the client, keep side conversations between you and the interpreter to a minimum. Advise the interpreter to request clarification from you or the client as needed. Pause frequently when speaking in session to give the interpreter sufficient time to interpret all that is being said.

The Intake Assessment

Ask About the Physical and Medical Symptoms of COVID-19

Prior to the start of treatment, obtain a history of the onset of the COVID-19 acute illness and treatment course, specific ongoing symptoms, current treatments, and any factors that improve or exacerbate symptoms. Identify and prioritize clients' specific areas of symptomatic concern. Some suggested language includes:

> *"I want to talk about the impact of COVID-19 on your life and ability to function as you'd like day to day, including any symptoms you may be struggling with. Are there specific concerns that you have about your health? What symptoms do you find particularly problematic, distressing, or interfering? What challenges have these symptoms presented to your daily life?"*

Assess the Client's Understanding of Their Medical Needs and Treatments

Clients may have trouble recalling all the details of their treatment team or physician recommendations. Also assess for lifestyle recommendations (e.g., increase physical activity, modify diet, quit smoking).

"Who is the primary medical provider for your treatment? What sort of recommendations did they make for your care? Were there any specialists or treatments they may have suggested during your last few visits? Along with the symptoms you mentioned above, have your providers mentioned any other concerns about your health or recommendations for your recovery?"

If the Client Was Hospitalized

Ask the client if they required hospitalization during the acute phase of COVID-19. If the client was hospitalized, ask about their discharge plan and treatment recommendations. Ask also about the client's length of stay in the hospital and whether mechanical ventilation or other invasive medical procedures were required. Explore how treatment has evolved since they contracted COVID-19. Gain an understanding of how the client views their current symptoms and their recovery expectations.

"How has treatment differed over the course of your recovery? Are you currently participating in rehabilitation, or has this been recommended to you? If so, what has your experience been like? How do you feel about your progress in rehabilitation so far?"

Medications

Ask about current medications, medication adherence, and availability of any equipment recommended (e.g., portable oxygen tank, pulse oximeter, blood pressure cuff).

"What medications are you currently taking? What are they for? Do you take them regularly? Over the past 2 weeks, how many days do you think you missed? Do you have any trouble getting medication refills? Have you ever missed a day, skipped a day, or taken your medications at times other than prescribed (late afternoon instead of the morning)? Do you know what condition your medications are intended to address?"

Normalize to clients that many individuals take medications without knowing what they are for; that's quite common, but having that knowledge can help clients make informed decisions about their care and recovery. Importantly, knowing the role or purpose of medications can also increase adherence to use.

Assessments

For Mood, Anxiety, and Adjustment

Assess anxious arousal, worry, depressed mood/depressive symptoms, and adjustment to their illness. Anxiety and depression are highly heterogenous syndromes and diagnostic entities and thus at times are challenging to assess, even aside from the context of COVID-19. Many clients with whom we developed this treatment approach would, according to criteria from the fifth edition of the Diagnostic and Statistical Manual of Mental Disorders (DSM-5), be classified as having an adjustment disorder with anxiety and/or depressed mood. Some clients meet criteria for a major depressive episode or generalized anxiety disorder. It is important that your intake interview assess for the psychological symptoms that arise in the context of COVID-19 symptoms, which will form the basis of your case conceptualization and working cognitive behavioral model. Differentiating between depressive symptoms, worry, and anxious arousal—though often co-occurring—can help you to decide how to prioritize the modules contained in this Therapist Guide.

- By *depressive symptoms*, we refer to low mood; loss of interest/pleasure; amotivation; guilt; poor appetite; disturbed sleep; feelings of worthlessness, helplessness, or hopelessness; and/or suicidal ideation.
- By *worry*, we refer to ruminative thoughts that for our clients may revolve around COVID-19 symptoms and their meaning. Worry is usually experienced as interfering with daily activities, over-whelming, and/or difficult to control.
- By *anxious arousal*, we refer to somatic, panic-type manifestations of anxiety experienced as an onset of fight-or-flight system activity such as shortness of breath, rapid heart rate, sweating, and other markers of physiological arousal.

Therapist Note

The above psychological symptoms, particularly anxious arousal, can overlap with physical/medical symptoms of COVID-19, and it can be difficult to disentangle one from the other. When physical/medical symptoms have an emotional component, (1) they are often experienced as more intense than would be suggested based on a client's medical status alone; (2) they may be associated with unhelpful thoughts and maladaptive behaviors; and (3) they are usually accompanied by other cognitive and affective symptoms and behaviors. Even if the cause of a physical/medical symptom is difficult to determine, if that symptom is accompanied by unhelpful thoughts and maladaptive behaviors, the thoughts and behaviors can still be targets of treatment. By addressing psychological factors that may exacerbate physical symptoms, clients may experience relief in both domains.

For Cognitive Difficulties

The following questions may be helpful in assessing for changes in cognitive function or symptoms of "brain fog," which can inform use of the module that targets these symptoms (Chapter 9). It can also be helpful to administer a self-report measure of cognitive difficulties such as the Patient-Reported Outcomes Measurement Information System (PROMIS) cognitive function scale (Saffer et al., 2015).

"Have you noticed any difficulties in thinking, concentrating, or memory? Does it take longer than it used to for you to complete tasks? Does your thinking feel slowed down? Are you less organized than you used to be? Do you feel easily overwhelmed by information? Is it challenging for you to multitask? Do you have trouble remembering words or names? Is it hard for you to remember events, names, or details from the recent past? Is it hard for you to remember to do things in the future, such as take a medication at a certain time or remember upcoming doctors' appointments?"

For the Functional Impact of Anxiety and Depression After COVID-19

The client's adjustment difficulties and anxiety and depressive symptoms may impact everyday function. These symptoms can impede the client's participation in valued activities. Assessing discrepancies between the consequences of anxiety or mood symptoms (e.g., avoidance, isolation) and the client's goals (e.g., to be a reliable parent, to be an efficient coworker) can help motivate clients to address maladaptive behaviors using the strategies in this program.

For Resiliency and Adaptive Coping Strategies

Ask about strategies, systems, or environmental modifications that the client has made to attempt to manage the physical/medical symptoms of COVID-19. Assess the impact (and helpfulness) of these strategies. We also recommend assessing resilience factors and positive emotions. Chapter 3 contains examples of positive emotions that clients can experience after COVID-19. This will allow you to gain a more complete picture of the client's psychological functioning in the context of a life-altering illness.

For Cultural Identity, Barriers to Care, and Preferences

Explore the client's cultural identity and examine how cultural factors impact presenting problems, views on mental health, and sources of support for the client. Drawing from Hays's (2008) multidimensional approach to assessing cultural identity, we recommend considering various aspects of the client's identity and background, including such factors as age and generational influence, nationality, citizenship, race, ethnicity, indigenous heritage, geographic region/environment, socioeconomic status, gender, sexual orientation, developmental and/or acquired disabilities, religious affiliation, and spirituality.

Screening for Suicidal Ideation and Contraindications for Participation in This Treatment Program

Suicidal Ideation

It is important to assess for suicidal ideation, intent, plan, and history of suicidal behaviors. Suicide risk assessment can help you manage suicide risk and create a safety plan and can be a consideration in referring the client for a higher level of care. We recommend use of the Columbia Suicide Severity Rating Scale, a validated, evidence-based, and freely available suicide assessment instrument.

Psychosis

If your client presents with signs and symptoms of a psychotic disorder—such as hallucinations or delusions—we recommend referring for a higher level of care, as this treatment program was not developed for use in individuals with psychosis. Note that hallucinations and delusions can be a symptom of delirium in clients who are hospitalized or who have acute metabolic disturbances or infections. Delirium is a transient state that typically resolves over time with delirium management protocols.

Substance Use

When assessing for the presence of substance use, it is important to do so in a matter-of-fact, non-biased manner that conveys a nonjudgmental attitude and allows clients the space to be forthcoming about their use. Characterizing the type of drug or alcohol used, frequency, duration of use, and related functional impact can help you understand whether the client's use is problematic. Our treatment program was also not developed for individuals with primary alcohol or substance use disorders. Framing substance use as a potential initial treatment target can be met with defensiveness; thus, referring the client for such treatment may be more effective if conveyed in the spirit of Motivational Interviewing while validating the client's presenting mood symptoms. For example, you may say:

"I see that you are experiencing emotional distress that requires follow-up care, and you may be trying to cope in both helpful and unhelpful ways. If I may suggest, it may be best to first work on decreasing your use of substances and then look again for mood symptoms, as [name of drug/alcohol] can sometimes make mood difficulties worse. I will provide you with a referral to a clinician who specializes in working with

individuals who actively use substances, and you can choose how you would like to proceed."

Severe Cognitive Impairment and Dementia

This treatment program can be implemented with individuals with mild cognitive impairment. Chapter 9 provides tools and strategies to help clients manage mild cognitive difficulties and symptoms of "brain fog" after COVID-19. Individuals with severe cognitive impairment/dementia who require assistance for activities of daily living, and/or whose pre-existing cognitive disorder has been worsened by COVID-19, will likely need specialized intervention and will not be appropriate for this treatment program. Referral for a neuropsychological assessment can help characterize the extent and severity of cognitive impairment and may inform decision-making and treatment planning.

PTSD

Clients with a primary diagnosis of PTSD may benefit from evidence-based psychotherapy for PTSD such as prolonged exposure or cognitive processing therapy. PTSD can occur in individuals who have experienced medical trauma (i.e., clients hospitalized in intensive care units). Therefore, it is important to assess for signs and symptoms of PTSD as part of the initial assessment, especially in clients who were hospitalized with severe symptoms of COVID-19. Even clients who were not hospitalized may have increased risk for developing PTSD if they have experienced traumatic events (i.e., witnessing the death of loved ones or working on the frontlines with patients who were critically ill). The PTSD Checklist 5 (PCL-5), a validated self-report tool (Blevins et al., 2015), is a brief instrument that can be useful for PTSD screening.

Self-Report Measures and Symptom Tracking

Administering periodic self-report measures of psychological symptoms can be a useful tool for symptom tracking. Self-report measures can also guide case conceptualization and supplement information obtained in the initial clinical interview. At the onset of treatment, self-report of symptoms can help determine the nature, frequency, and severity of the client's psychological distress; provide valuable information about targets for change; and help therapists prioritize treatment modules. For example, a client endorsing severe anxiety and distress with physiological arousal/tension may benefit from an initial focus on relaxation strategies. When selecting self-report measures, it is important to consider their applicability (constructs assessed are valuable and can guide therapy), practicality (brief, easily accessible, cost-efficient, and easy to score and interpret), and psychometric properties (validity, reliability, sensitivity to change). When developing and implementing this program, we used the Hospital Anxiety and Depression Scale (HADS) for clients treated in the hospital. For clients treated in the community, we used the 9-item Client Health Questionnaire (PHQ-9) and the 7-item Generalized Anxiety Disorder Questionnaire (GAD-7).

Cultural Considerations and Adaptations to Treatment

This section of the introduction provides an overview of culturally responsive care to clients from culturally diverse backgrounds. We discuss the importance of culture in the context of therapy, provide a brief overview on current and historical trends that impact ethnic minority communities, and introduce concepts and strategies that promote culturally responsive care when working with clients with COVID-19. Our goal is to provide practical tools to adapt treatment approaches for enhanced clinical care of ethnoculturally diverse populations. Two optional worksheets (A: Cultural Identity Questionnaire and B: Cultural Values and Relevant Experiences) are provided in the Appendix at the end of this guide to help you further assess and explore your client's cultural identity, values, and beliefs. These worksheets can help inform how the client's cultural perspectives and culture-specific stressors influence their clinical symptoms and engagement in treatment. Those two worksheets can also be accessed by searching for this book's title on the Oxford Academic platform, at academic.oup.com.

Cultural Identity

Culture encompasses a system of values and norms that shape life experiences, belief systems, and the way we navigate the world. In the context of therapy, culture can influence an individual's perspective on mental health and illness, trust in healthcare providers, communication styles, treatment preferences, and outcomes.

Culture in the Context of COVID-19

"Culturally responsive treatment delivery" has become the gold standard of care and has been mandated by a large majority of professional mental health organizations (American Psychiatric Association, 2016; American Psychological Association, 2017; National Association of Social Workers, 2015). The demand for culturally informed care grew in response to research highlighting racial and ethnic disparities in mental health access, quality of care, and treatment outcomes.

Appeals for culturally responsive care became even more salient in the wake of the COVID-19 pandemic, which had a disproportionately negative impact on ethnic minority communities and further highlighted inequalities across racial, ethnic, and socioeconomic groups. As compared to their White counterparts, ethnic minorities had higher rates of COVID-19 infection and disease severity (Khunti et al., 2020; Magesh et al., 2021) and significantly higher prevalence rates for mental illnesses including depression, suicidal ideation, and substance misuse following the pandemic (McKnight-Eily et al., 2021). The overrepresentation of ethnic minorities experiencing illness, loss, and hardship throughout the pandemic was a stark reminder of the racial trauma that continues to impact these communities.

In conceptualizing your client, we recommend that you explore the many intersections of a client's cultural identity, with a specific emphasis on strengths and resilience experienced on the individual and community level. Consider also systemic and sociopolitical factors that may be influencing the harsh but often overlooked realities experienced by clients of color, such as racism, oppression, immigration concerns, and poverty. Below are some considerations to make when working with culturally diverse clients with persisting symptoms of COVID-19.

Therapeutic Alliance

Building Rapport and Trust

It is important to consider the client's cultural preferences and worldview to determine the most effective way to foster rapport and trust in the therapeutic relationship. Individuals from certain ethnic minority cultures may find it difficult to relate to therapists who conduct themselves in an impersonal and business-like manner (Brown et al., 2015). Although interpersonal preferences vary across cultures, warm and personal approaches that include judicious self-disclosure are often preferred to cultivate trust and therapeutic alliance in the first session (Fung & Lo, 2017; Organista, 2006; Taylor et al., 2006). Questions pertaining to family stigma, gender roles, and discrimination—which may reflect unfavorably on the client's culture and family/loved ones—can be addressed after establishing sufficient rapport in therapy (Paradis et al., 2006). This is particularly true in cross-cultural contexts when the client identifies with a minority and/or underrepresented culture and the therapist presents as a member of the dominant culture. In this context, the client may be reluctant to disclose sensitive information to the therapist out of concern that it may reinforce and perpetuate stereotypes and prejudices against individuals of their cultural community (Hays, 2009).

Cultural Humility

Cultural humility is an interpersonal stance that emphasizes interpersonal sensitivity; genuine curiosity; and willingness to honor the values, beliefs, and customs of another person. It involves an ongoing process of self-awareness and self-evaluation, in which therapists routinely examine and become aware of how their cultural background and biases impact treatment. This interpersonal stance promotes openness to learning about the cultural perspectives of the client and having them inform you of their values rather than making erroneous assumptions based on stereotypes.

A common error is to assume that racial and ethnic similarities between client and therapist are indicators of a shared culture and worldview. Reducing the concept of culture to racial and ethnic minority status can discount the nuanced complexities and richness of a client's culture. Additional aspects of cultural humility that you can practice include:

- Seeking to neutralize power imbalances that may arise between you and the client
- Acknowledging that you are susceptible to making mistakes
- Communicating to your client that they should correct you if a misunderstanding arises in treatment.

The Appendix at the end of this Therapist Guide contains case vignettes highlighting concepts in cultural considerations as well as two optional worksheets. Case Vignette 1 (see pages 235–237) is a brief illustration of how to practice cultural humility in session.

Culturally Informed Case Formulation

Presenting Complaints

Culture influences the way we view and express emotions, manifest symptoms of distress, attribute explanations to our conditions, and set goals. For example, a client who identifies with collective values may want to prioritize addressing symptoms that have a significant impact on the overall well-being of the family as opposed to symptoms that are more exclusively distressing for the client. Culturally informed questions that may be helpful in guiding the clinical interview include:

"How do your family or members of your community view your concerns? What do they attribute these difficulties to? Do you share similar perspectives on these issues? If not, what do you believe to be causing your difficulties?"

Cultural Strengths and Supports

Identify cultural strengths and supports that can be incorporated into treatment. Explore cultural supports across multiple levels of the client's surrounding environment, including home/family, religious/spiritual community, and demographic community. Common examples of supports include family cohesion, access to resources, prayer or meditation, and culturally specific artistic expression such as ritual dance, music, and art.

Client-Relevant Goals and Treatment Planning

In Chapter 1, we discuss goal setting. When working on goal setting with your client, having an understanding of their cultural identification and values can help identify goals that are meaningful to the client and may capture culturally specific goals that you otherwise may not have known. Consider whether the desires and expectations of family and/or the broader community influence the client's goals and expectations. Explore the client's preference for family involvement and cultural customs, from a nonjudgmental stance that does not pathologize their preferences. Lastly, incorporate personally held values into the client's goals and treatment plan. Ask the client if they have any preferences or cultural convictions they would like to include in therapy, such as prayers or rituals.

Addressing Common Cultural Barriers to Change

Illness Attribution

Clients with strong beliefs about the medical etiology of their psychological distress may be reticent to engage in behavioral interventions and may feel that medical intervention is the only solution to their condition. In these cases, it may be helpful to (1) validate the client's experience; (2) discuss the interplay between physical and mental health conditions that often coexist among clients with COVID-19-related illness; and (3) provide psychoeducation about the potential physical and mental health benefits of behavioral intervention, which is often helpful in normalizing, validating, and increasing willingness to engage in treatment. However, if the client continues to be resistant to behavioral intervention and demonstrates limited interest in continuing treatment, it may be helpful to provide them with referrals for psychiatric treatment (psychopharmacological intervention).

Religious and spiritual attributions to mental illness are common among many ethnic minority cultures and often surround moral judgment from a higher power, retribution for previous misdeeds, and/or misfortune imposed by supernatural forces. Clients with such attributions may feel overcome with guilt and lack the motivation to engage in therapy. Similarly, a client who identifies with devout religious and spiritual traditions may believe that prayers and sacraments or rituals will heal them from their ailments, and that participating in therapy may be construed as a lack of faith in the higher power in which they believe. In these cases, it is best to acknowledge the religious and spiritual perspectives of the client while simultaneously exploring the potential costs that arise from their inactive participation in treatment. The client may become more amenable to therapy if elements of their religious/spiritual faith are incorporated into treatment (e.g., religious contemplative practice as part of mindfulness or relaxation exercises, behavioral activation that incorporates spiritual or religious activities).

Stigma

Mental health stigma is a common barrier to treatment across cultures. Mental illness and treatment can be viewed as an indictment of one's character and construed as a sign of personal weakness. The stigmatization of the individual may also extend to their relatives or loved ones. Oftentimes, being affiliated with an individual diagnosed with a stigmatizing mental illness can jeopardize the family's reputation, social status, and relationships with members of their community. As such, an individual diagnosed with a stigmatizing mental illness may not only face derision from members of the broader community but may also be susceptible to experiencing a sense of guilt or shame for dishonoring the reputation and social status of their family and/or community. Some family members may also experience a sense of guilt and responsibility for the individual's condition, especially among families who deem mental illness to be an outgrowth of poor parenting or lack of familial support. Over time, individuals may begin to give credence to the stigma prevalent in their communities and espouse negative beliefs about their own self-worth, self-efficacy, and abilities (Balsa & McGuire, 2003; Clement et al., 2015, Hudson, 2005).

When examining the impact that stigma may potentially have on a client, it may be helpful to ask:

"How is mental illness and treatment viewed in your culture? How are individuals with mental illness typically treated in your community? How does stigma concern you, if at all? Does mental illness bring shame to the family and/or community? If so, can you describe how that impacts them and how this may affect you?"

Destigmatizing mental illness and therapy early in the treatment process can help strengthen the therapeutic relationship and enhance willingness to engage in treatment. To destigmatize mental illness, begin by normalizing the client's psychological distress and discuss the ubiquity of human suffering. Educate the client on how anxiety, depression, and adjustment difficulties are very common in individuals with both acute and chronic medical conditions, including COVID-19. Note that psychologists and social workers are increasingly embedded within medical care teams, highlighting the importance and recognition of mental health as a component of COVID-19 care. This can assuage the isolating experience and negative self-appraisals that often arise with seeking mental health care. In our experience, encouraging clients to consider their anxiety and depression in the context of the global suffering incurred by the COVID-19 pandemic, or as an understandable response to their intensive medical hospitalization/treatment and persisting COVID-19 symptoms, was helpful in normalizing and destigmatizing both psychological distress and therapy. For clients who are reluctant or feel uneasy about terms such as "mental illness" and "therapy," it can be helpful to frame the treatment program as a way to develop new skills to better manage their COVID-19 symptoms.

Acculturative Stress and Family Expectations

Acculturation refers to the dynamic process of assimilating to a new, oftentimes dominant culture, while simultaneously sustaining contact with native culture. The acculturation process can be a psychological and socially stressful transition (Umaña-Taylor et al., 2009), and it is common for generational differences between family members to exacerbate this stress due to divergent values and expectations among them (Fanfan & Stacciarini, 2020). Consider how the acculturation process may be contributing to your client's psychological distress and/or engagement in treatment. Case Vignette 2 (Appendix, pages 237–238) provides a brief illustration.

Discrimination and Internalized Oppression

If your client identifies as a member of an underrepresented group or ethnic minority communities, ask the client about any experiences of discrimination, particularly in the healthcare and medical setting. If the client reports experiencing discrimination, ask them how these experiences have shaped their self-view, view of others, and ways of navigating the world. Examine if the client has internalized harmful beliefs about themselves, and over time, help them recognize the damaging implications these beliefs may have on their behaviors, values, and goals as it relates to adjusting to the persistent symptoms of COVID-19. See Case Vignette 3 (Appendix, page 238) for an example.

Culturally Informed Adaptations for Specific Skills in This Treatment Program

Reframing Unhelpful Thoughts

Questioning the accuracy of thoughts or beliefs during cognitive restructuring can be invalidating and may even be perceived as evidence of the therapist's lack of cultural understanding and/or sensitivity. Rather than challenging the accuracy of thoughts, ask the client whether thoughts are *helpful* and consistent with the client's values.

Behavioral Activation

Incorporate activities that are culturally relevant and meaningful to the client, particularly those that may foster a sense of interconnectedness with the client's culture and community. This could include engaging in religious/spiritual services, playing culture-specific instruments and music, engaging in artistic expression that is consistent with their heritage, or becoming involved in social justice groups that advocate for their community. Be mindful of potential financial concerns, family obligations, work/school demands, and flexibility, which may potentially impede engagement in scheduled activities.

Mindfulness

Religious and spiritual perspectives should be considered when introducing mindfulness in treatment. Although it can be helpful to present mindfulness as a practice that is distinct from any religion or spiritual faith, many clients may still view its practice as being inextricably linked to Buddhism and resist applying this technique because it violates their faith. It is helpful to clarify misconceptions clients may have about mindfulness (and to note that meditative practice has been used over the course of many centuries in almost all religions). It may also be helpful to incorporate experiential mindfulness exercises as opposed to meditative practices, as this may be less threatening/concerning to the client as a religious practice that runs counter to their spiritual beliefs (i.e., mindful walking and mindful eating). If the client continues to be reticent to try mindfulness practices, be respectful of those preferences and incorporate other techniques that may facilitate mindful practice. Alternatively, the client could use meditative practice that incorporates elements of their own belief system (i.e., religious scripture, holding religious emblems/figures while praying).

Adherence to Medications

Clients with poor health literacy may not fully understand the implications of misusing or discontinuing prescribed medications. For example, some clients may adhere to medications when symptomatic and discontinue them when symptoms abate; this pattern is worth exploring with clients as it may contribute to inconsistent remission of symptoms and worsening mood, anxiety, and frustration. In the same vein, ethnic minority communities more often use herbal and homeopathic remedies for their medicinal properties and are less inclined to report use of these alternative remedies to their treating physicians (Gardiner et al., 2013). While we want to encourage clients to honor cultural traditions, we also want to emphasize how critical it is that they report their use of homeopathic and herbal remedies to their prescribing physicians to avoid potential contraindications.

Relatedly, fears of addiction and/or lifelong reliance on medications are reported among ethnic minority communities and may contribute to poor adherence to prescribed medication regimens (Nicolaidis et al., 2010). Provide a space for the client to share their concerns. Validate their experiences and fears, and encourage them to express their concerns to their physician. If the client expresses feeling insecure or having difficulty communicating their concerns to their prescribing physician, you can use behavioral techniques (role reversal, rehearsal, role-play) to enhance the client's interpersonal approach and assertiveness. This may also strengthen their confidence in advocating for their needs when working with providers. An example of what this may look like is illustrated in Case Vignette 4 (Appendix, page 239).

Loss and Grief

COVID-19 mortality rates were highest in ethnic minority communities that are likely to also be disproportionately impacted by loss and grief (Liu & Modir, 2020). Explicit and implicit rules for grieving, communal gatherings, and commemorating the lives of those lost vary across cultures and were disrupted by the COVID-19 pandemic. For example, communal gatherings were largely restricted, which impacted how individuals were able to connect with other community members around grief. Culturally specific grieving behaviors, customs, and rituals—and the ways they were and continue to be impacted by the pandemic—should be considered when treating clients grieving the loss of loved ones. Cultural customs and ritual elements can be incorporated into treatment and may include practices such as meditation, symbolic communication with the deceased (e.g., drumming ceremony, commemorative ceremony), and symbolic expression (e.g., moment of silence at the start of an activity, writing assignments or poems, use of religious or spiritual text). These customs and rituals may require modification depending on any ongoing restrictions on gathering.

As noted earlier in this introduction, two optional worksheets (A: Cultural Identity Questionnaire and B: Cultural Values and Relevant Experiences) are provided in the Appendix to help you further assess and explore your client's cultural identity, values, and beliefs. (Note that these two worksheets do not appear in the Client Workbook. They are meant for the therapist to guide the client in completing, if needed, and not for the client to self-administer.) Alternatively, assessment forms and client worksheets can be accessed by searching for this book's title on the Oxford Academic platform, at academic.oup.com.

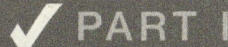

PART I

Skill Building

CHAPTER 1

Module 1: Setting Goals for Therapy

Chapter Overview

The purpose of this chapter is to introduce approaches to facilitate goal setting and enhance motivation in treatment. Worksheet 1.1: Goal Setting and Worksheet 1.2: Processing Pros and Cons are provided to assist in this process.

Number of Sessions

The recommended number of sessions for this chapter is one, although a second session can be helpful to clarify goals for clients who may have difficulty articulating goals and/or have suboptimal motivation. If you find that clients are "stuck" about change throughout the course of treatment, refer back to this chapter to help resolve ambivalence. While there is not a formal assigned at-home practice in this chapter, you should encourage your client to reflect on and refine/adapt goals that are set in session.

Therapeutic Content

Motivation

Motivation to engage in therapy is essential to initiating and maintaining behavioral change. For many clients, motivation will vary throughout treatment, and bolstering motivating factors early on can help to address natural fluctuations in motivation throughout the course of treatment

(Barlow et al., 2017). Goal setting is one of the most effective ways to foster motivation and achieve behavioral change. Goals provide a clear focus for treatment, help inform and direct therapeutic interventions, and improve the likelihood of successful behavioral change. Along with approaches to formulate treatment goals, this chapter integrates strategies from Motivational Interviewing (MI), a collaborative, evidence-based approach designed to foster internal motivation (Martins & McNeil, 2009; Miller & Rollnick, 2012; Palacio et al., 2016).

Goal Setting

Begin by obtaining a general sense of the client's goals or desires for treatment. For example:

"What brought you into treatment? How do you hope that I might be able to help you? What are you looking to get out of treatment? How would you like for your life to be different a few years from now?"

Then, introduce Worksheet 1.1: Goal Setting in session to help review specific concerns or mood/anxiety symptoms that prompted the client to seek treatment and the impact of reported symptoms on the client's life. Worksheets can be found at the end of this chapter in both the Therapist Guide and Client Workbook or can be accessed by searching for this book's title on the Oxford Academic platform, at academic.oup.com. The initial questions on the worksheet can be explored together in session with the client and help to prioritize symptoms and concerns and to develop long-term goals. Collaborate with the client to develop two or three long-term goals and write them down (or type them out if you are conducting a telehealth session). Next, help the client break the long-term goals into short-term goals. Use the "SMART" framework to help the client articulate and write (or type) goals that are specific, measurable, achievable, relevant, and time-bound. Setting realistic and achievable goals improves the chance of attaining these goals. Formulating measurable goals provides both clients and therapists with an objective understanding of treatment progress and gains. The process of breaking long-term goals into short-term goals (intermediate steps) can make goals more specific, measurable, and achievable. If a goal is too vague or general, the prompts on Worksheet 1.1 can be useful to add specificity and delineate specific short-term goals.

Barriers Impacting Goal Setting

Some clients may be bogged down by perceived obstacles, which can make it difficult to isolate and establish goals. For clients responding to questions about goals by communicating concerns about barriers, direct the conversation by saying, "Let's talk first about where you want to go, before we consider how to get there." Other clients may be focused on a physical goal ("I want to be able to run a 5K again") where attainment is largely out of your direct purview as a therapist. In such cases, explore how the client's thoughts and emotions may be impacting their approach toward that goal and attempt to reframe the goal in a way that incorporates the impact of mood and anxiety ("I want to better manage my anxiety so it does not get in the way of training for the 5K"). Finally, some clients may have goals about "eliminating" or "getting rid of" anxiety, low mood, or certain thoughts and fears. For reasons the client will learn in Chapter 3, such emotions cannot be eliminated entirely. Thus, you will want to reframe the goal for the client to be more realistic—for example, reducing the frequency or intensity and increasing the ability to manage (but not eliminate) an emotion.

Involving Others

Goal setting may involve consultation and support from care partners. Family members and loved ones can be an essential resource in helping the client formulate goals, particularly if the client is from a cultural background in which family-based or community-oriented goals are important. For clients with a higher level of disability or those who have difficulty functioning independently in specific domains, goals may require the assistance and support of care partners. With the client's permission, it can be helpful to work with the client and their loved ones to develop treatment goals.

> **Therapist Note**
> *The long-term durability of persistent symptoms of COVID-19 is still largely unknown and treatments continue to be developed as of the time of writing. Depending on the severity of their initial illness, some clients may not be able to return to their previous level of functioning. The extent of potential gains may be unclear or may evolve over time. Identifying goals that are not achievable can lead to resignation, hopelessness, and treatment dissatisfaction. Consultation with the client's medical providers can offer a clear view of the client's limitations and prognosis, which can help to set attainable goals and identify specific targets for treatment. Emphasize realistic, stepwise change, and help to shape goals that are manageable and accommodate the client's disability and limitations.*

Enhancing Motivation and Resolving Ambivalence

MI approaches can be helpful early in treatment to explore and strengthen internal motivation for change, particularly for clients with ambivalence (Miller & Rollnick, 2012). There are two key components of motivation. The first is a wanting or desire to change, and the second is self-efficacy or confidence in the ability to achieve change. Building motivation is difficult if the client believes change is out of reach for them. Some clients may recognize the benefits of change but lack confidence that they can make the change happen. The strategies below, adapted from Miller and Rollnick (2012), are designed to help resolve ambivalence and foster motivation by invoking the client's own desire and capacity for change.

Eliciting Internal Motivation for Change

Evidence suggests that people become more committed to what they hear themselves express or say aloud. The following prompts and discussion points are designed to help clients articulate their own specific desires and reasons for change and provide an opportunity to express aloud their internal motivations:

> *"What do you wish for in your recovery? How would you like for things to be different? What don't you like about the way things are now? If you*

were successful in fully engaging in treatment, how might your life be different (6 months from now, 5 years from now?) What's challenging about the way things are now? What could be some advantages of [addressing X symptom]? If you did make this change, what could be different? What would be the best outcome? How urgent or significant does this feel to you? How important is it for you to make this change?"

Importance Ruler

The "importance ruler" is a strategy that encourages the client to articulate why change is important, and it provides helpful information about how important the client feels it is to address this concern. To use this tool, say to the client:

"Now that we have a sense of your goals, let's talk a bit more about why they're important to you and how you feel about addressing them. On a scale from 0 to 10, where 0 means 'not at all important' and 10 means 'the most important thing for me right now,' how important would you say it is for you to address [this symptom/treatment goal]?" (Miller & Rollnick, 2012, p. 175)

The answer will be a number between 0 and 10. Even if the client provides a low number, this presents an opportunity to elicit or evoke personal reasons for change. Once the client responds, follow up by asking, *"Why are you a '2' and not a '0'?"* Although unusual when beginning treatment, a client may respond with an importance of "0." This would indicate no ambivalence and little current desire for change. Further approaches to enhance motivation, particularly in the context of the client following their medical treatment plan, are outlined in Chapter 11.

To further explore any ambivalence, consider using Worksheet 1.2: Processing Pros and Cons as an optional in-session exercise. The worksheet can help ascertain sources of ambivalence and maladaptive beliefs or assumptions that can be addressed in treatment. Discussing the pros and cons of changing helps to identify potential barriers and factors that may influence engagement or motivation. This exercise also helps to build motivation by encouraging clients to generate reasons against staying the same and in favor of making a change. Remember that worksheets can be found at the end of this chapter in both the Therapist Guide and Client Workbook or can be accessed by searching for this book's title on the Oxford Academic platform, at academic.oup.com.

Assessing and Strengthening Confidence and Self-Efficacy

Evaluating Self-Efficacy

The following questions are designed to assess the second important element of motivation—the client's self-perceived ability to achieve the desired change. Refer to Chapter 11 for additional strategies.

> *"What do you think you might be able to change? How confident do you feel that you could pursue this change, if you chose to do it? Of the various areas of concerns and goals we've discussed, which seem most possible or addressable?"*

Fostering Confidence: Confidence Ruler

The "confidence ruler" strategy allows you to quantify the client's perceived confidence and self-efficacy, and identify ways to enhance the client's confidence to pursue the desired change. To use this tool, ask the client:

> *"How confident are you that you could do this if you decided to? On a scale from 0 to 10, where 0 is not at all confident and 10 is extremely confident, where would you say you are?"* (**Miller & Rollnick, 2012**)

Explore any responses that are lower than a 10. Gain a sense, from the client's perspective, what might help increase their sense of self-efficacy and how therapy can facilitate this. For example, ask, *"What would it take for you to go from a 2 to a 5? How might I help you go from a 2 to a 5?"* This enables the client to help generate ideas and identify specific ways to improve their sense of confidence in pursuing their goals. In addition, elicit from the client their own strengths and sources of confidence: *"On the other side of the coin, tell me why you are a 2, and not a 0?"*

Enable the Client to Generate Internal Solutions

Confidence can be increased by exploring personal sources of strength and providing opportunities for the client to generate internal solutions to potential obstacles (Miller & Rollnick, 2012, pp. 219–221). Explore the client's own thoughts for how best to pursue their goals and address potential obstacles. Allow the client to serve as a source of ideas. This can provide a roadmap to barriers and potential solutions, and helps to strengthen the client's sense of ability and capacity for change. For example:

"If you decided to pursue this change, what would that look like? Given what you know about yourself, and the difficulties you've overcome in the past, how could you successfully make this change? What are some strategies you could use to get started? What could be a good first step? What obstacles do you foresee? How might you be able to address them?"

Leverage Past Experiences

Assess difficult changes the client has made in the past or stressful events they have overcome. This can accentuate the strengths and skillsets that are already present within the client and encourages the client to identify and articulate them. Elicit specifics on how the client made that change. Reflect strengths and qualities raised in the discussion, particularly those that may be generalized to the current circumstance:

"What changes have you made in the past that were difficult for you? Have there been other times when you experienced a sudden medical or physical illness and were able to recover? What was most helpful for you in that situation? Have there been times when you felt like you wouldn't be able to do or accomplish something, but were eventually able to? What have you been able to do that you weren't sure at first you could do? Why did you decide to make that change? What did you do that worked, or that you found most helpful? What obstacles did you run into, and how were you able to overcome them?"

Coordination of Care with Medical Providers

Most medical and rehabilitation providers have a shared goal: to improve client independence, everyday function, and well-being. Coordination of care with medical providers can be vital to achieving optimal client outcomes. Communicating directly with medical providers can have a meaningful impact on client recovery and help define important areas of focus for treatment.

Obtain permission from the client to contact their primary care provider, specialty provider (e.g., cardiologist, pulmonologist), and/or rehabilitation therapist to discuss their medical regimen and needs. Your contact with providers will largely occur outside of session. At initial contact, explain that you are providing mental health services to your shared client. Emphasize that you know the impact of emotions and mental health on physical function and medical illness, and you would like to incorporate in treatment ways to maximize uptake and engagement with the provider's medical recommendations. Listed below are several advantages and areas of focus for discussions with medical providers:

- **Gain an understanding of the client's medical needs, limitations, and prognosis.** Obtaining a clear view of the client's progress and prognosis can help to set realistic goals and ensure treatment strategies are personalized to the client's specific needs and abilities. In addition, assess for any concerns the medical provider may have about the client's adherence to treatment recommendations. This can reveal areas of difficulty with medical engagement that can be targeted in treatment to advance client recovery.

- **Facilitate coordination of care across specialties.** Poor coordination of care among medical providers can worsen treatment outcomes. For some clients, all providers may be within one hospital system and will therefore have access to the client records and treatment progress across specialties. However, other clients may receive treatment from providers at different clinics. This may put more of the onus on the client to provide updates from one provider to another, which can often be difficult. In our experience, clients who have been through COVID-19-related illness report being overwhelmed by the number of clinicians with whom they follow up. As a therapist building a comprehensive understanding of your client's care, you can help bridge these specialties by direct communication with providers as indicated. The specialist may also share other resources available to the client that were previously unknown, like community or medical center resources (e.g., support groups, exercise programs, recreational services).

■ **Arrive at a synergistic and targeted approach for adherence enhancement if the client's mental health symptoms are interfering with adherence to medical care.** Medical providers recognize the importance of medical treatment but may not be aware of how the client and family respond to treatment recommendations. In addition, providers may be unaware of the client's mental health symptoms, or how these symptoms can influence treatment engagement. Once you have a clear view of the providers' role and specific concerns, provide them with a brief summary of the client's symptoms and their impact on behavior and treatment engagement. Depending on the medical providers' domain, you may also establish a collaborative plan to address client adherence. For example, if the client has a fear of falling that is impacting their ability to progress in physical therapy, jointly plan with the client's physical therapist to coordinate therapeutic interventions. Establish concrete approaches to integrate and reinforce strategies introduced in sessions (e.g., self-soothing, grounding exercises) into physical therapy visits.

Therapist Note

Some clients who come to you may not have had a full medical workup, nor be actively under the care of relevant medical specialists. During the intake and goal-setting process, if it becomes clear that the client has had no or minimal medical follow-up, then we recommend referring to relevant medical providers. At a minimum, your client should be under the care of a primary care physician or internal medicine physician. If your client has physical difficulties, mobility limitations, or pain, then referral to a physiatrist (a rehabilitation medicine physician) can be helpful. Relatedly, a physical therapy referral should be considered if your client is experiencing physical difficulties, mobility limitations, dysautonomia (dizziness, vertigo), or breathing difficulties. If your client presents with neurocognitive symptoms and/or fatigue, then referral to a neurologist can be beneficial. Many specialty clinics for post-acute COVID-19 or "long COVID" now exist and can be options for care depending on the client's geographical location.

At the end of your goal-setting session, explain to the client that at home practice will be an important part of this treatment program. Research has shown that in cognitive behavioral interventions such as this one, greater out-of-session practice is associated with greater treatment gains. Though this first goal-setting session does not have a formal at-home practice, encourage your client to spend time reflecting on their goals and thinking about whether they need to be refined. Explain to your client that as they reflect, they may want to expand on their goals and the pros/cons exercise below at home on their own.

Worksheet 1.1
Goal Setting

> **Instructions:** Select 2-3 goals for treatment that you value and are important to your well-being. Use this worksheet to specify both major or long-term goals and short-term or intermediate steps you can take to achieve them.

Begin by identifying **long-term goals** for treatment. Using the prompts below, consider the most pressing or important symptoms or concerns you'd like to address in treatment.

- *What symptoms do you find particularly problematic, distressing, or interfering?*
- *What challenges have these symptoms presented to your daily life?*
- *How would you like for things to change?*
- *What would you like to see improve?*
- *What do you hope treatment could help you address or accomplish?*

Then, identify several **short-term goals** or intermediate steps that you can take to work toward each of your long-term goals. To come up with short-term goals, break each long-term goal into pieces until each part is concrete and measurable. Identify specific behaviors, activities, and experiences that would indicate progress toward your long-term goal. Short-term goals should fit the **SMART criteria**, listed below. For each short-term goal, provide as many details as you can, including how, when, and in what timeframe you plan to achieve them. For instance, how will you track your progress? What will you use to measure your progress? How will you know you've achieved your goal? How long will it take you to achieve your goal?

The SMART Criteria

Specific. What is the specific action, event, or outcome you'd like to achieve?

Measurable. How will you measure your progress or success?

Achievable. Are your goals doable and realistic? Are they too lofty?

Relevant. Are the goals meaningful to you, or personally relevant or significant? Does your short-term goal fit in with your values and long-term goal?

Time-bound. What is the time period for accomplishing this goal?

```
┌─────────────────────────────────────────────────┐
│                Long-term Goal                   │
│                                                 │
│ ─────────────────────────────────────────────── │
├─────────────────────────────────────────────────┤
│                Short-term Goals                 │
│                                                 │
│ ─────────────────────────────────────────────── │
│                                                 │
│ ─────────────────────────────────────────────── │
│                                                 │
│ ─────────────────────────────────────────────── │
│                                                 │
│ ─────────────────────────────────────────────── │
└─────────────────────────────────────────────────┘


┌─────────────────────────────────────────────────┐
│                Long-term Goal                   │
│                                                 │
│                                                 │
│                                                 │
├─────────────────────────────────────────────────┤
│                Short-term Goals                 │
│                                                 │
│ ─────────────────────────────────────────────── │
│                                                 │
│ ─────────────────────────────────────────────── │
│                                                 │
│ ─────────────────────────────────────────────── │
│                                                 │
│ ─────────────────────────────────────────────── │
└─────────────────────────────────────────────────┘
```

Worksheet 1.2
Processing Pros and Cons

This worksheet can be used to help you figure out the advantages and disadvantages of making
a desired change versus staying the same, so you can determine the choice that's best for you.
Use the questions and prompts below to help you consider the advantages and disadvantages
of making a change, and then make a decision about your next steps.

PROS	CONS
Of Changing	Of Changing
Of Not Changing	Of Not Changing

Taking Stock of the Big Picture

- If your symptoms of depression or anxiety were better, how would life be different? What would you do first? Think about how this might look in different areas of your life (at work, at home, and in your relationships).
- Looking toward the future, how would you like things to change or be different than they are now?
- Think for a moment about a loved one or family member. What do you think their goals might be for your well-being or recovery? What do you think they might feel about you making this change? Why do you suppose they would feel this way?

Pros of Changing

- If you did make this change, what could be different? What would be the best possible outcome? How could this change impact your quality of life, well-being, or recovery? Try to be as specific as you can.
- What are some good things that could happen or result from making this change? How do these results align with your goals for your treatment or recovery? How about your values, the things that are most important to you?
- Look toward the future. If you are successful in making this change, how might your life be different 6 months from now, 1 year from now, and 5 years from now?
- If your symptoms were reduced by 20%, how would this feel? How could life be different?

Cons of Not Changing

- What worries you most about this symptom, in the long run?
- Even if you don't envision this happening to you, what might be some potential consequences for someone who doesn't make this change?
- What might be the downsides of not making this change?

Making a Plan to Pursue Change

- Were there other times you faced a sudden illness or other sudden change in your life? What was that like? How did you respond?
- What changes in your health have you made in the past that were difficult for you?
- Why did you decide to make that change then? How did you go about doing it? What did you do that worked, or that you found most helpful?

- Have there been times when you felt like you wouldn't be able to do or accomplish something, but were eventually able to?
- Given what you know about yourself, and the difficulties you've overcome in the past, how could you successfully make this change now?
- What are some strategies you could use to get started? What might be a good initial step?
- Are there others (family, friends, loved ones) who you could call on for support? In what ways could they be helpful? If you hit a roadblock, how might they be able to help?

CHAPTER 2

Module 2: Covid-19 and the Cognitive Behavioral Model

Chapter Overview

The purpose of this chapter is to (1) provide the client with education on COVID-19; (2) introduce a cognitive behavioral model of anxiety and depression after COVID-19; and (3) discuss how physical/medical symptoms of COVID-19 and associated thoughts, emotions, and behaviors contribute to difficulties in everyday functioning, and limit engagement in and adherence to medical interventions. The client starts to track symptoms, thoughts, emotions, and behaviors. Two worksheets are used: Worksheet 2.1: Cognitive Behavioral Model and Worksheet 2.2: Tracking Thoughts, Emotions, and Responses to COVID-19 Symptoms.

Number of Sessions

One to two sessions are recommended. In the first session, focus on providing psychoeducation and an introduction to the cognitive-behavioral therapy (CBT) model. In the second session, review the CBT model and introduce self-monitoring, which is assigned for at-home practice (homework). Depending on client uptake, a third session can be spent on reviewing the CBT model and self-monitoring. Consider administering self-report symptom questionnaires (e.g., PHQ-9, GAD-7) at the beginning of the session to track symptoms of depression and anxiety.

Providing Education on COVID-19 Using the "Elicit–Provide–Elicit" Framework

Knowledge and understanding of COVID-19 illness and treatment may vary widely from client to client. It is important to first gain an understanding of what the client knows about COVID-19 and their medical treatment, before educating or providing information. Use the "elicit–provide–elicit" sequence of information exchange (Miller & Rollnick, 2012). This is a collaborative and stepwise approach to psychoeducation that first assesses the client's understanding and areas of concern and helps to prioritize the discussion on those areas most important to the client. This approach can increase openness and receptiveness to the information provided.

1. **Elicit.** At this point, after your intake interview, coordinating with the client's medical/rehabilitation provider(s), and goal setting, you should have a good idea of your client's COVID-19 symptoms, medical recommendations, and treatment plan. Review and elicit the client's current understanding of the etiology and treatment of COVID-19 symptoms. Eliciting first provides a template of the client's current understanding and allows you to identify any gaps in knowledge and areas of focus to target in treatment:

   "Tell me what you know about COVID-19 and how it can affect people. Tell me what you already know about [client's treatment] and how it works. Tell me what you already know about what factors contribute to or worsen your COVID-19 symptoms. Tell me what your doctor has told you about your recovery and prognosis."

2. **Provide.** Provide psychoeducation, using the information contained in this chapter and any up-to-date research or public health information. Start by asking the client what information they want or need about their COVID-19 symptoms and treatment. This is a collaborative approach that enables the client to direct the discussion and communicate what would be most helpful to them. Asking first emphasizes the client's autonomy and can help increase receptiveness to the information provided:

"I wonder if I might be able to tell you some things that I've noticed with other people who have felt anxious or depressed after COVID-19, had difficulty adjusting to persisting COVID-19 symptoms, or have found their recovery was slow/unsatisfying? There has been some interesting new research on [symptom of treatment] post-COVID-19. Would you mind if I tell you a bit about it? Some people have asked me about [symptom or treatment]. Would it be alright if we discussed this for a few minutes? There's another piece that I notice we haven't discussed yet. Can we focus on this for a few minutes?"

3. **Elicit.** Elicit the client's understanding of the psychoeducation provided, as well as their thoughts and reactions to the information provided. Assess for clarity and any persistent questions or areas of misunderstanding.

"So, what do you make of that? What do you think? Does that make sense so far? How does your experience fit in with the information we just discussed? Could I explain that better? How does that sound? What else would you like to know about [area of concern]?"

Education on COVID-19

The following education on COVID-19 is likely to be important to introduce, at a minimum:

- The World Health Organization (WHO) and the medical and scientific community all recognize that symptoms of COVID-19 can persist after the initial infectious period.
- COVID-19 symptoms and the affected parts of the body are highly heterogenous and vary from person to person.
- COVID-19 symptoms can persist from the initial illness, but may also present after an initial recovery.
- Symptoms can wax and wane, with good days and bad days.
- COVID-19 symptoms, particularly during or immediately after the infectious period, may or may not persist in the long term. This is an important distinguishing factor because it can help clients to mitigate any catastrophizing of normal recovery processes. This is particularly important for hospitalized clients and those who were recently discharged to the community.

▪ We do not yet know what might cause symptoms of COVID-19 to persist. Leading hypotheses actively being studied include ongoing immune activity and inflammation, cardiovascular effects of the virus, changes to the endocrine system that regulates hormonal activity, and persistence of viral remnants in the body. Because symptoms of COVID-19 are highly variable, it is likely that there is more than one cause for persistent symptoms, and that these cause(s) differ from person to person. The uncertainty surrounding persisting symptoms of COVID-19 can be highly frustrating and anxiety-provoking for many clients. We find it helpful to validate this uncertainty and the accompanying emotions it can bring.

▪ Despite the uncertainty regarding a definitive cause for persistent symptoms, the *emotional experience and suffering* (i.e., the symptoms of anxiety and depression) following COVID-19 are treatable. Further, by treating anxiety and depression, some clients notice improvement in their physical symptoms as well—though this is by no means a guarantee. Regardless of improvement in physical symptoms, alleviating anxiety and depression can improve quality of life, facilitate better management of COVID-19 symptoms, improve engagement in medical and self-care, and improve function at home and at work.

Therapist Note

Throughout this discussion, it is not necessary for you to know or come up with all the right answers. There are some questions you may be able to answer. Many others, such as those pertaining to specific medications or medical specialties, may be beyond the scope of your expertise. There is no pressure or expectation to answer questions outside of your area of knowledge. Encourage the client's thoughtfulness, discernment, and commitment to their care. For such questions, provide a general response and defer to their medical providers for additional information. Clients will appreciate your honesty. Write the question down in session and recommend that they pose it to their medical provider(s) during their next visit. If it is a more immediate concern that's impacting their care, treatment, or health, encourage them to reach out and schedule an appointment, and help the client troubleshoot this process, as needed.

Psychoeducation on COVID-19 and Thoughts, Emotions, and Behaviors

Reiterate to the client that the goal of this treatment program is not to alleviate, eliminate, or treat the medical/physical symptoms of COVID-19; rather, the goal is to help the client better manage their symptoms, cope with distressing thoughts and emotions, engage in adaptive behaviors, and live a life of meaning consistent with their values. To illustrate the association between COVID-19 symptoms and thoughts, emotions, and behaviors, start by showing your client the cognitive behavioral model in Figure 2.1.

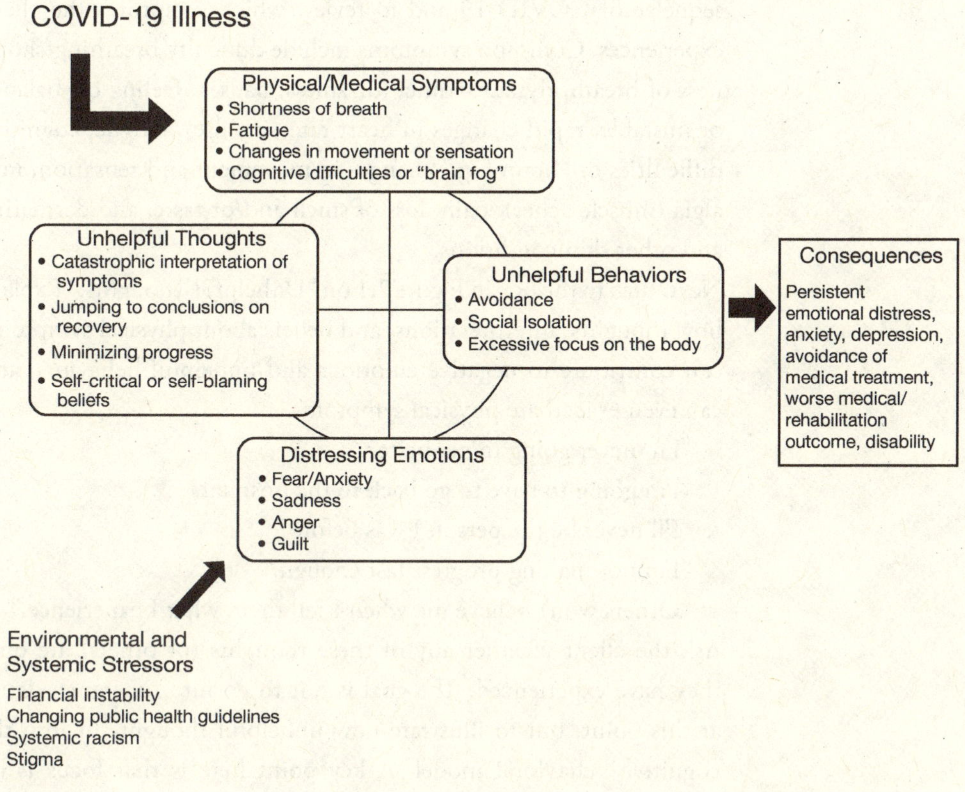

COVID-19 Illness

Physical/Medical Symptoms
- Shortness of breath
- Fatigue
- Changes in movement or sensation
- Cognitive difficulties or "brain fog"

Unhelpful Thoughts
- Catastrophic interpretation of symptoms
- Jumping to conclusions on recovery
- Minimizing progress
- Self-critical or self-blaming beliefs

Unhelpful Behaviors
- Avoidance
- Social Isolation
- Excessive focus on the body

Consequences

Persistent emotional distress, anxiety, depression, avoidance of medical treatment, worse medical/rehabilitation outcome, disability

Distressing Emotions
- Fear/Anxiety
- Sadness
- Anger
- Guilt

Environmental and Systemic Stressors

Financial instability
Changing public health guidelines
Systemic racism
Stigma

Figure 2.1.

A Cognitive Behavioral Model of Thoughts, Emotions, and Behaviors and Their Association with COVID-19 Symptoms

As an overview of the model, emphasize that COVID-19 can result in persisting physical/medical symptoms, which can trigger unhelpful thoughts, distressing emotions, and maladaptive behaviors. These thoughts and behaviors in turn exacerbate the sequelae of COVID-19 and contribute to persistent emotional distress, avoidance, worse medical outcomes, and disability.

- Start with the box in Figure 2.1 that refers to "Physical/Medical Symptoms," which is often the easiest for clients to describe and is most closely related to COVID-19 itself. As part of the intake assessment, you should have some working knowledge of the predominant physical/medical symptoms experienced by the client. Nonetheless, it can be helpful here to review the most common sequelae of COVID-19 and to review which symptoms the client experiences. Common symptoms include difficulty breathing/shortness of breath, dysautonomia (dizziness, nausea, feeling off-balance or unstable, rapid changes in heart rate or pulse), fatigue, cognitive difficulties or "brain fog," changes in movement and sensation, myalgia (muscle aches), pain, loss of smell and/or taste, and dermatitis and other skin conditions.
- Next, turn to the box in Figure 2.1 on "Unhelpful Thoughts." Explain how thoughts, interpretations, and beliefs about physical symptoms can contribute to negative emotions and unhelpful behaviors, and can even exacerbate physical symptoms.
  - "I'm never going to get better."
  - "I'm going to have to go back to the hospital."
  - "I'll never be the person I was before."
  - "I'm not making progress fast enough."
  - "Others won't believe me when I tell them what I experience."
- Ask the client whether any of these thoughts (or others) are ones they have experienced. The goal is not to go into too much depth at this point, but to illustrate how unhelpful thoughts fit into the cognitive behavioral model. A key point here is that focus is on the *helpfulness* (and unhelpfulness) of thoughts. Some catastrophic reactions to symptoms of COVID-19 do include classic thinking traps (discussed in more detail in Chapter 7). However, many clients with COVID-19 face an uncertain prognosis and course with the possibility of long-term and chronic sequelae. Thus, clients' beliefs about the persistence and impact of their COVID-19 are not always

distorted. However, those thoughts may still be contributing to anxiety and depression, interfering with medical care, and impacting everyday function. Thoughts that may have truth to them can still be unhelpful and contribute to maladaptive behaviors, leading clients to be "stuck" in a cycle of negative emotions and maladaptive behaviors.

- Next, turn to the box in Figure 2.1 labeled "Distressing Emotions." Explain how physical/medical symptoms of COVID-19, as well as unhelpful thoughts, can trigger emotions that are experienced as uncomfortable, distressing, or intolerable. These emotions can include fear, anxiety, sadness, anger, embarrassment, shame, guilt, frustration, and demoralization. Point out that any of these emotions can occur in the context of COVID-19. Emotions can be distressing in their own right and can fuel further negative thoughts and maladaptive behaviors.

- Then, turn to the box in Figure 2.1 labeled "Unhelpful Behaviors." As in classic cognitive behavioral models, point out behaviors in response to physical/medical symptoms, emotions, and thoughts that can seem helpful (adaptive) in the short term but typically have negative (maladaptive) consequences in the long term. The following maladaptive behaviors can occur in the context of COVID-19:

  - **Avoidance:** Clients often avoid situations that they fear may exacerbate (psychological or physical) symptoms or that make symptoms subjectively intolerable, avoid follow-up appointments and medical care because of a fear of receiving bad news, avoid situations in which their symptoms or limitations are apparent to others, and avoid experiencing distressing emotions (sadness, grief, anxiety) that are perceived as unwanted or unbearable. Although avoidance can lead to a reduction in emotional intensity and physical symptoms in the short term, in the long term it often perpetuates anxiety and depression, worsens disability, and restricts participation in medical care and valued activities.

  - **Social isolation:** Social isolation can be conceptualized as a form of avoidance. It can be helpful to discuss it separately here given its prevalence and its association with depression. Clients with persisting sequelae of COVID-19 may isolate themselves from their community, family, friends, and loved ones. They may do this because they perceive social interaction as potentially exacerbating physical symptoms and distressing emotions. They may also isolate because of anxiety about social judgment, stigma, potential neurocognitive deficits or physical changes, or in general how they may be perceived by others. In the long term, social isolation can perpetuate depression and reinforce feelings of inadequacy or disability.

■ **Excessive body focus and vigilance to physical symptoms:** In response to ongoing physical symptoms, or novel and/or unusual bodily sensations, clients can engage in excessive focus and be overly vigilant to bodily sensations. For example, a client may excessively check their oxygenation using a pulse oximeter. A client may repeatedly check to see if a limb moves as it should. A client with symptoms of brain fog may test their memory repeatedly out of fear they may lose information. And a client may be on guard as to whether a certain movement or activity exacerbates any ongoing sensation. While focusing on the body can provide reassurance and/or a sense of control in the short term, it reinforces the notion that physical sensations cannot be tolerated and keeps the client on guard to threat.

The Impact of the Cognitive Behavioral Cycle

The impact of the cycle of unhelpful thoughts, distressing emotions, and maladaptive behaviors is to perpetuate anxiety and/or depression. Define both anxiety and depression for the client:

■ Anxiety is characterized by concerns and worries, typically about the future, that one perceives as overwhelming and difficult to control. Sometimes the worries can become so intense that they disrupt sleep and contribute to muscle tension. Anxiety can also be experienced physiologically as shortness of breath (hyperventilation), rapid heart rate, sweating, and gastrointestinal distress—these symptoms can come on rapidly akin to panic attacks. In many clients with COVID-19, the physiological symptoms of anxiety overlap with the sequelae of COVID and can be difficult to distinguish.

■ Depression is characterized by persistent depressed mood; loss of interest or pleasure in daily activities; loss of motivation; poor self-esteem; loss of appetite; sleep disturbance; feelings of worthlessness, helplessness, guilt (which in COVID-19 can manifest as the client perceiving they are a burden on caregivers), and hopelessness; and suicidal ideation. Psychomotor slowing, fatigue, and sleep disruption are also symptoms of depression. In some COVID-19 clients, these "bodily" symptoms of depression (fatigue, insomnia) can overlap with the physical symptoms of COVID-19 and are difficult to distinguish.

Like other psychiatric disorders, the presence of anxiety and depression after COVID-19 and whether it is conceptualized as warranting treatment depends on its frequency, intensity, and interference in everyday function. That is, depression is more than just being sad, and anxiety is more than just feeling worried. Symptoms are experienced as intense, persist over time, and interfere with the client's daily life.

The Impact of Environmental and Systemic Stressors

At the time of writing this Therapist Guide, multiple additional stressors have emerged during the COVID-19 pandemic and are currently ongoing. New viral variants continue to be documented and reported. Rates of infection, hospitalization, and death continue to ebb and flow. Public health guidelines at the national and local levels continue to shift. All these factors create uncertainty. Highlight to the client that uncertainty and unpredictability are important drivers of anxiety. The toolbox of skills learned in this treatment can also help the client manage the uncertainty and stress of the pandemic.

Economic hardship and uncertainty persist for many. Systemic racism and structural inequalities came to the forefront during the acute phase of the pandemic with findings that Black and Hispanic Americans suffered disproportionate effects of COVID-19. With the murder of George Floyd in 2020 and the protests that followed, many began to frame the COVID-19 pandemic and systemic racial injustice as twin pandemics. Be aware of the role environmental and systemic stressors can play in the client's experience of COVID-19. Validate the role of environmental and systemic factors in contributing to the client's difficulties. Acknowledge the impact of these factors and the difficulty in effecting structural change, which can lead to a sense of powerlessness, hopelessness, and resignation. Instead of attempting to change these factors, emphasize that the goal of treatment is to help the client to best function in the context of their unique environment and stressors. The toolbox of skills learned can help the client better cope with and manage the stress of structural contributors to stress, anxiety, and depression.

A Client Example of the Cognitive Behavioral Model

Once you have gone over the cognitive behavioral model, use the sample cognitive behavioral model provided in Figure 2.2 to illustrate a typical example of a client's experience with COVID-19, including associated thoughts, emotions, behaviors, and consequences.

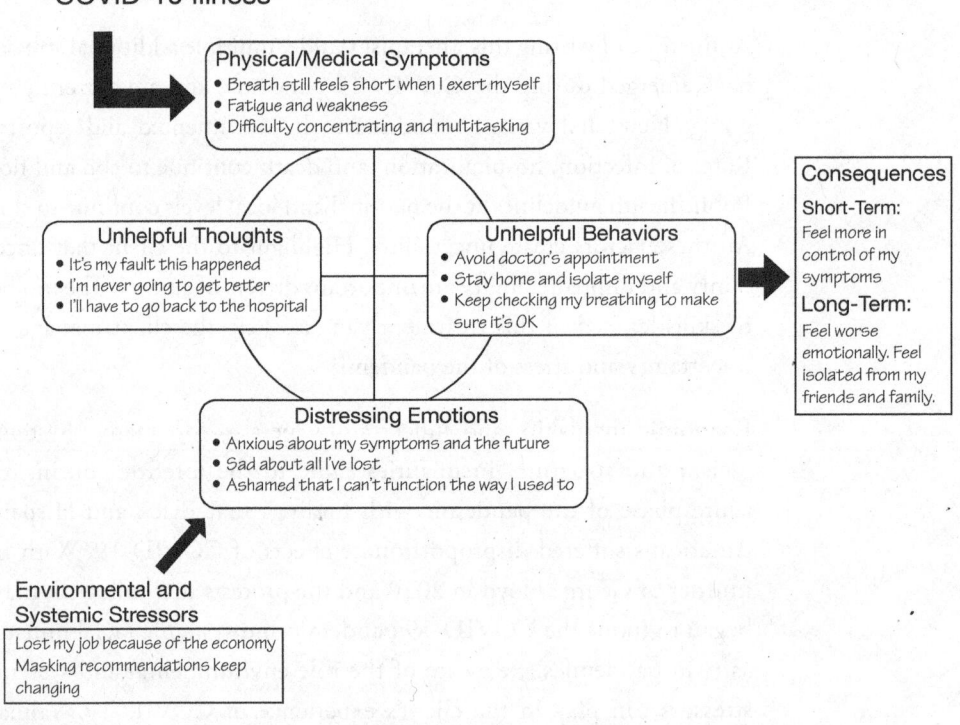

Figure 2.2.

Marta's Completed Cognitive Behavioral Model Worksheet

In session, use Worksheet 2.1: Cognitive Behavioral Model, and fill out an example specific to your client. This worksheet can be found at the end of this chapter in both the Therapist Guide and Client Workbook or can be accessed by searching for this book's title on the Oxford Academic platform, at academic.oup.com. Anchor the client to a specific experience, activity, or event in the past week. Explore the specific thoughts, emotions, and behaviors that arose. Discuss any systemic or environmental factors that may have contributed to the client's response. Finally, explore what happened afterward in the short term and the long term. How did the client feel, think, or act? Did the symptoms get better or worse? Did the client's thoughts and behaviors bring them closer to leading the life they want? Did their thoughts and behaviors help them to engage in the medical care important for recovery?

At-Home Practice

As discussed in the Introduction to this Therapist Guide, at-home practice is a critical ingredient of treatment success. Review with your client the importance of practicing skills outside of session. Note that research on cognitive behavioral interventions such as this one has shown that homework completion is beneficial for treatment gains. Problem-solve with your client any potential barriers that they anticipate for at-home practice completion. If your client is resistant to completing homework, it may be helpful to use Worksheet 1.2: Processing Pros and Cons, specifically for homework completion (see Chapter 1) or to break down the task. For example, you can suggest that your client fills out at least three different examples using three copies of Worksheet 2.1: Cognitive Behavioral Model over the next week (rather than one each day). For at-home practice, provide the client with additional blank copies of Worksheet 2.1, and ask them to fill out examples as they occur throughout the week. This worksheet can help the client think through the relationships between thoughts, emotions, and behaviors. In the subsequent session, use Worksheet 2.2, which is a consolidated version of the model in a table format and allows the client to jot down experiences more quickly as they arise.

Worksheet 2.1
Cognitive Behavioral Model

COVID-19 Illness

Physical/Medical Symptoms

Unhelpful Thoughts

Unhelpful Behaviors

Distressing Emotions

Environmental and Systemic Stressors

Consequences
Short-term:

Long-term:

Worksheet 2.2

Tracking Thoughts, Emotions, and Responses to COVID-19 Symptoms

Situation	COVID-19 symptom	Thoughts	Emotions	Behaviors (What did I try to manage the situation?)	Consequences

CHAPTER 3

Module 3: Identifying and Understanding your Emotions after Covid-19

Chapter Overview

The purpose of this chapter is to provide the client with a framework for emotion awareness and identification in the context of persisting symptoms of COVID-19. Topics covered include identification and labeling of emotions, as well as helping clients learn to self-validate emotional responses to COVID-19-related illness and sequelae. Two worksheets are incorporated: Worksheet 3.1: Emotion Myths (used to help clients identify their own emotion "myths" or unhelpful attitudes around emotions) and Worksheet 3.2: Catching Emotions Rising (practice exercise to help clients identify and label their emotional experience and triggers).

Number of Sessions

One to two sessions are recommended for this content. For clients who quickly grasp the concepts and/or are familiar with psychoeducation on emotions, one session may be sufficient. Identifying and validating emotional experiences related to COVID-19 illness using the material in this and subsequent chapters can be revisited in future sessions, as needed. Consider administering self-report symptom questionnaires (e.g., PHQ-9, GAD-7) at the beginning of the session to continue tracking symptoms of depression and anxiety.

COVID-19 can contribute to emotional distress among those with persisting symptoms, many of whom may not have previously experienced a similar intensity or chronicity of unpleasant emotions. Emotions that are adaptive to an extent in the context of medical illness—including fear, sadness, anger, and guilt—may become maladaptive if they interfere with a client's ability to adjust to the chronicity of symptoms or changes in the way they navigate their environment. Difficulties identifying, understanding, and tolerating unpleasant or painful emotions may contribute to unhelpful thoughts and maladaptive behaviors that interfere with illness recovery. Individuals with persistent physical/medical symptoms of COVID-19 infection may experience intense and often unpleasant emotions as a result.

Addressing emotional distress includes psychoeducation and validation of emotional responses as well as increasing your client's awareness of their attitudes and beliefs toward emotional distress (emotion myths). Recognizing and labeling emotions is an important first step for the emotion regulation techniques contained in the following chapters. Labeling, understanding, and self-validating emotional experiences can decrease the intensity or "temperature" of emotional experiences themselves. It can bolster the client's sense of agency and demystify what can be a confusing or unfamiliar experience. We have found that psychoeducation and validation of emotions is among the most helpful tools to use with clients recovering from COVID-19.

The following case vignette illustrates how emotions and beliefs about emotions may manifest in the context of COVID-19, as well as the role of psychoeducation and validation of emotions. Case vignettes and sample session scripts are provided throughout chapters to illustrate key concepts and therapeutic techniques. Case vignettes and sample session scripts that illustrate principles of culturally informed care are provided in the Appendix.

Case Vignette 3.1

Mr. Jones is a 68-year-old man who has never been in therapy. After he contracted COVID-19, he underwent a lengthy hospitalization. After being treated for the acute infection over several weeks, he was physically weak and had to go to inpatient rehabilitation before being discharged home. He experienced intense anxiety when he was told he would have to stay in the hospital longer than he expected. He was unfamiliar with and unsure of what was happening to him, as his thoughts were catastrophic, and he felt as if they were spiraling.

After discharge from the hospital, Mr. Jones was referred for psychotherapy. Initially, he identified emotions of fear, shame, guilt, and grief that were sudden and so intense that he thought he was "going crazy." He thought that if he talked about his feelings they would "take over" and he would never feel like himself again. Mr. Jones reported that he was raised to not talk about feelings, and his dad would often tell him to "man up." The therapist provided psychoeducation on the evolutionary function of all feelings and the adaptive value that fear and grief have in the context of COVID-19. Mr. Jones and his therapist worked together to identify situations when experiencing certain unpleasant feelings was valid versus when these feelings did not fit the situation. Through clarification of his emotional experience, and identification of the emotion myths that were holding him back from accepting and experiencing his emotions fully, he began to feel less guilt and shame and began to accept his feelings as valid and even manageable.

Defining and Identifying Emotions

Start by going through Figure 3.1: Identifying Difficult Emotions with your client in session. This figure (which appears in both the Client Workbook and this Therapist Guide) provides a brief description of why emotions exist and the adaptive function that each emotion serves. It also provides common physiological manifestations for each emotion. For some clients the somatic (bodily) sensation may be an important cue for identifying emotions.

In the session, go through each emotion and explore to what extent the client has experienced it in the context of COVID-19.

Fear/Anxiety	Sadness	Anger/Frustration
• Fight-or-flight "alarm" system that warns us of danger or threat and helps us plan for future problems • Physical manifestion: rapid increase in heart rate, sweating, rapid and shallow breathing, restlessness, tension	• Helps us grieve and process loss, and signal to others we need help • Physical manifestation: decreased energy, tearfulness	• Helps us stand up for ourselves and others in response to wrongs, injustice, or blocked goals • Physical manifestation: increase in heart rate and blood pressure, fluhsed face
Disgust	**Guilt**	**Shame**
• Helps us distance from or reject an object, event, or situation that is potentially contaminating or offensive • Physiological manifestation: nausea, upset stomach	• Helps motivate us to make amends, communicate remorse, and repair a social violation • Physiological manifestation: low mood, tightness in chest or "lump" in stomach	• Motivates us to withdraw because a behavior is perceived as offensive to the community, particularly if a social norm has been violated • Physiological manifestation: low mood, tightness in chest or "lump" in stomach

Figure 3.1.

Identifying Difficult Emotions

Below are examples of how emotions may manifest in the context of COVID-19:

1. **Fear/Anxiety**: During the acute illness phase, fear may have motivated the client to pay attention to symptoms that needed to be brought to medical attention. Fear may have also motivated behaviors such as masking that are geared toward minimizing infection. After the acute infectious phase, or in times of relatively low viral transmission, fear may occur even if there is not an immediate threat and therefore represents a false alarm. Similarly, some anxiety, closely related to fear, can be helpful to motivate your client to be cautious and vigilant around medical precautions, for example a client whose motor function has been impacted and needs to be more careful when walking to prevent falling. Clients may feel some anxiety that motivates them to prepare for a medical appointment or to plan for travel. However, anxiety can be unhelpful when it is disproportionate to the situation, is distressing, or leads to avoidance.

2. **Sadness:** Clients may feel sadness because of lost bodily function, lost goals, lost time (due to illness/hospitalization), death of loved ones, and changes in work or family roles. Some sadness can help the client grieve and process these disruptions. However, if sadness becomes intense or persistent or interferes with daily functioning, it can be maladaptive and result in depression.

3. **Anger/Frustration:** Anger may occur toward societal structures and systems that failed in the pandemic response. Anger can also occur toward individuals the client sees as not taking COVID-19 or related precautions seriously. Anger can even be a response to physical or emotional pain. Clients may feel anger or frustration when thinking that they never should have gotten sick, that they were not listened to or treated properly (medically), or that their friends or loved ones don't understand their experience and how painful it has been. Anger can motivate the individual to stand up for themselves and rectify perceived wrongs. However, the chronic experience of anger can lead to alienation from interpersonal relationships, conflict, and a sense that the client is drifting from their own sense of values.

4. **Disgust:** Disgust may be felt by clients whose environment does not align with their values of protecting their own health or the health of loved ones. For example, some clients may feel that infection prevention measures (masking) align with their value system and subsequently experience disgust when faced with people who decide not to wear masks or get vaccinated.

5. **Guilt:** Clients may feel guilty that they should have done something to prevent their own infection or the infection of someone else. They may feel "survivor's guilt" if they survived their illness but a loved one did not. They may feel guilty about being unable to function as they did prior to COVID-19, particularly if a spouse or family member has had to take on extra responsibilities or provide aid or support to the client. Some guilt can motivate a repair in interpersonal relationships or reflections on how the client can adapt and still contribute to a family or community. Excessive guilt, however, can be paralyzing and exacerbate depression.

6. **Shame:** Similar to guilt, clients may believe that they should have been able to overcome the illness or that they never should have "allowed themselves" to be exposed to begin with. Some clients may

believe that they should be able to overcome what they are feeling with "willpower." These beliefs can contribute to clients feeling like they are "broken" or "defective," and they may even point to evidence of not being able to work anymore or contribute to prior household roles in the same way. They may report feeling like they want to avoid others, may avert their gaze when talking to the therapist or to other people, and may feel embarrassed with social contact.

You can use the discussion above to begin to discuss with clients when the emotions "fit the facts" (i.e., are congruent with the situation or trigger) by discussing common scenarios that warrant different types of emotional responses. Note that the emotions above, particularly the "negative" emotions, may all be adaptive, particularly if they helped the client get through the acute phase of their infection/illness. However, emotions may become maladaptive if they lead to avoidance behavior, are overly intense or distressing, and/or no longer "fits the facts." If clients are having trouble identifying what they would feel in a situation, encourage them to tell you what they think a friend or loved one would feel. You can also suggest that they reflect on any physiological or bodily changes and possibly even thoughts and behaviors (see Chapter 2) for cues as to the emotion present.

Identifying if an emotion "fits the facts" can also be difficult if the client experiences secondary emotions. Secondary emotions are emotional responses to an initial emotion. For example, if your client becomes angry with their doctor before a visit, it may be a secondary emotional response, with the primary emotion being fear of bad news or rehospitalization. Work with the client to break down the specific thoughts, sensations, and feelings they had over the course of the event. Disentangling emotion responses and acknowledging and validating the primary emotion can be helpful in reducing emotional distress.

As part of this exercise, go through Figure 3.2: Identifying Positive Emotions (which appears in both the Client Workbook and this Therapist Guide), and ask the client if they have experienced any of the following positive emotions over the course of their recovery and rehabilitation from COVID-19. Clients with persisting symptoms of COVID-19—despite suffering from negative emotions that are intense and distressing—also experience positive emotions such as happiness,

Happiness	Gratitude	Inspiration
• Focuses us on enjoying activities that enhance pleasure and pursuit of personal/social values	• Helps acknowledge growth and change and communicate appreciation to others	• Inner feeling of being moved, sometimes in response to new information, in a way that motivates us to act or pursue an endeavor

Determination	Curiosity	Pride
• Feeling of inner strength that helps us to persist in the face of challenges	• Focuses our attention on people, events, or information that may be beneficial to us	• Inner sense of accomplishment that helps us acknowledge our gains and contributions

Figure 3.2.

Identifying Positive Emotions

gratitude, inspiration, determination, curiosity, and pride. Having clients identify such emotional experiences can draw out their inner resilience and can also convey the important idea that multiple emotions can be experienced at the same time. A client might feel anxious about their COVID-19 symptoms and proud of what they accomplished in their last physical therapy session. They may be very afraid of what the future holds and experience determination to do everything they can to recover. Amidst significant adjustment difficulties, clients may have moments when they are able to feel happy and grateful. Note that for many, the idea that multiple emotions can be experienced simultaneously may be novel and should be normalized.

Dispelling Emotion Myths

Clients may have little experience with the degree of emotional distress they are experiencing following COVID-19 and may believe that unpleasant emotions are something to be feared or avoided. They may report feeling as if they are "going crazy" and judge themselves for not being able to "pick up the pieces and keep going."

After discussing the emotions above, it is often helpful to gently probe for the presence of such "emotion myths." The rationale for this is that emotion myths can be barriers to change and to self-validation of emotional experiences. Client beliefs that some emotions are "bad," unbearable, or even selfish can invalidate the client's emotional experience in the context of the threat of illness and lead to secondary emotions (guilt, shame) and further perpetuate suffering. Some clients believe that "willpower" should be able to overcome emotions. Others may believe that emotions are permanent rather than temporary. Some clients may believe that if they call attention to their unpleasant emotional experiences by exploring them, the emotions will spiral out of control.

Use Worksheet 3.1: Emotion Myths in session, to help clients identify which myths resonate, and provide psychoeducation on emotions to challenge these myths. It may be helpful to also discuss with clients the ways in which emotions were handled by their family systems in childhood as clients may be carrying internalized schemas of emotional experience and expression that become magnified and maladaptive in times of high stress or illness. Allow the client to explore these myths, including why they may be present, for example familial or cultural factors. Explore what might be a more helpful way for the client to think about emotions. Worksheets can be found at the end of this chapter in both the Therapist Guide and Client Workbook or can be accessed by searching for this book's title on the Oxford Academic platform, at academic.oup.com.

Self-Validating Emotional Experiences

Finally, introduce self-validation as an approach to facilitate emotional awareness and ultimately emotion regulation. By self-validation, we refer to noticing and labeling emotions with an added component of self-compassion. This can be difficult for clients who may feel that their emotions are not justified or who desire to avoid or get rid of them. It is important to point out that self-validation does not mean approval, liking, or wanting to feel a certain way. It simply means for the client to be open to what they are feeling. Explain to the client that self-validation of emotions can turn down the "temperature" (intensity) of the emotion and lead to more effective management of emotions using skills that will be introduced in future chapters. It can also lessen the potential for secondary emotions or emotions about emotions—that is, feeling embarrassed, ashamed, guilty, or weak for having a certain emotion.

Explain to the client that over the next week, as they track their emotions, they should attempt to add self-validation to emotion identification and awareness. Clients can self-validate by *describing*: labeling emotions and any associated physiological sensations while attempting to be as nonjudgmental as possible. Clients may say to themselves, "I'm feeling scared" or "I'm crying" while acknowledging the difficulty of their experience: "This has been really hard, and it makes sense I would be scared." Clients can also note how the emotion makes sense in terms of their experience with COVID-19: "Given that I suddenly ended up in the hospital with COVID, it makes sense that I still feel scared." "I've lost so much time being sick, it makes sense that I would feel sad." Clients can also note how an emotion is understandable given the current context or situation: "It's understandable I would feel angry after today's doctor appointment. My doctor was so rushed and didn't seem to have time for my questions."

Case Vignette 3.2

THERAPIST: *From what you have told me, Ms. Sanders, you certainly have been through a lot of ups and downs the last few months, trying to regain some of your physical functioning and strength.*

CLIENT: *Yeah, it has been a year since all that, and I just can't seem to shake it off, you know?*

THERAPIST: *Tell me a little bit more about what you mean.*

CLIENT: *Well, I just can't seem to get back to myself. I don't have the same energy, I am having trouble sleeping, and my mind just goes to the worst places, especially at night when I try to go to sleep. I toss and turn thinking about how my life changed and how I just can't seem to get it together. If I was strong enough, I would be able to shake it off and move on.*

THERAPIST: *It sounds like you went through a very difficult illness, one that altered your life in significant ways. If it's OK with you, can I share a little bit about what happens to our mood sometimes after serious illness, and specifically after COVID-19?*

CLIENT: *Sure.*

THERAPIST: *Well, there is a lot happening inside of our brains and bodies when we face a serious illness. In the battle to defeat the virus, our immune system goes on overdrive, our organs are stressed, and when you add to that the severity of illness that requires a stay in the hospital, well then our whole body and brain becomes taxed. The physical effects of that battle may be easy to see—people carry oxygen or walk with a cane—but there are also psychological effects that are harder to see. What do you feel?*

CLIENT: *I don't know, I am so turned around sometimes. Sometimes I think about the pain I caused my family seeing me in the hospital. And I was vaccinated, and I thought I was careful but maybe I wasn't. Maybe I should have been more careful. And now my family is suffering more because I can't work, I can barely play with my kids, and I am crying like a baby—I can't pull it together.*

THERAPIST: *Well, you may be feeling more than one thing, Ms. Sanders. It may be helpful to take a look at this list of emotions* [therapist points to Figure 3.1]. *Which emotions do you feel reflect what you are describing and experiencing?*

CLIENT: *I think sadness for sure. But also guilt. I have so much regret and sometimes it makes me angry but sometimes I just cry. And maybe a little shame? I mean, I am ashamed to be seen like this—blubbering with emotions—I can't hold it in.*

THERAPIST: *It sounds like you have identified several unpleasant feelings coming up, and that can feel emotionally overwhelming. I have noticed that you also may be pretty tough on yourself when it comes to feelings . . . have you noticed that yourself?*

CLIENT: *Well, I can't help it—what kind of a person cries all the time and can't support their family? My parents always told me to keep it together. If people see you cry, they will know you are weak and they will lose respect for you, and here I am crying all the time.*

THERAPIST: *What a tremendous burden you must feel, holding all of these painful emotions in and experiencing this much self-judgment for what is a very normal response to serious medical illness. We learn many ways to deal with our emotions from our family and throughout childhood. However, that does not always mean that we have to maintain the beliefs we form as children throughout our adult lives. How does it make you feel when you think to yourself you are weak for having emotions?*

CLIENT: *Terrible.*

THERAPIST: *Myths, or unhelpful beliefs we learn about our emotions, can have that effect. Take a look at some of the emotion myths that people commonly report. Can you indicate which ones ring true to you* [therapist points to Worksheet 3.1]?

CLIENT: *Well, pretty much this one and this one and this one down here. Wow, so you are saying these are all myths?*

THERAPIST: *People feel all sorts of feelings. Some we experience as painful and distressing and some are joyful or exciting, but they are all part of the human condition. There is no feeling that makes you a weak or strong person; there are just feelings. Our beliefs about what to do with those feelings can sometimes make us feel more pain as we try to push the feelings away or we judge ourselves harshly for feeling.*

CLIENT: *Yeah, that sounds like me. Every time I try to hold it in, I just end up feeling worse. So what do I do?*

THERAPIST: *Well, you have taken an important first step by identifying and labeling what you are feeling. What do you think about trying to practice identifying, labeling, and not judging your feelings for the week ahead?*

CLIENT: *I will give it a shot. Seems like it's worth exploring.*

At-Home Practice

Review with your client the importance of at-home practice. Assign Worksheet 3.2: Catching Emotions Rising. The goal of this worksheet is to have clients track their emotional experiences over the week along with the intensity and associated triggers. As part of this exercise, encourage your client to use self-validating statements as described above. When reviewing the worksheet during the subsequent session, start to explore with the client whether the emotion and the intensity of the emotion "fits the facts" or is disproportionately intense to the situation. For the former situations, remind the client of psychoeducation on emotions and why the emotion makes sense in that situation. If the presence of an emotion or its intensity does not "fit the facts," then the client can still validate the emotion as an understandable response, and you can note to the client that future sessions will focus on techniques to better regulate and manage emotions.

Worksheet 3.1
Emotion Myths

Emotion myth (place a checkmark next to those that apply to you)	What else might be true?
__"Feelings are for wimps"	
__"If I talk about my feelings I will make them real"	
__"Being [unpleasant feeling] means that I am a weak person"	
__"If I feel [unpleasant feeling] that is what I am meant to feel; I shouldn't have to work to change my emotional experience"	
__"Extreme emotions are the only way that people will take you seriously"	
__"Emotions come out of the blue and there is no way to manage them"	
___"Unpleasant emotions are bad and dangerous and should be avoided at all costs"	
___"If I am 'emotional' no one will take me seriously"	
___ "People only want to hear about happy feelings"	
___ "If I have strong feelings, I am out of control"	
___ "No one wants to be around a sad sap—I have to put on a happy face, otherwise I shouldn't even go out"	

Worksheet 3.2
Catching Emotions Rising

Take some time throughout the week to check in with your body, mind, and environment and try to identify and label what you are feeling. Use the last column to indicate the degree of intensity of your emotions.

Day/time	What were you doing?	Emotion	Intensity of emotion from 0 (absent) to 10 (most intense)
Monday			
Morning			
Evening			
Tuesday			
Morning			
Evening			
Wednesday			
Morning			
Evening			
Thursday			
Morning			
Evening			
Friday			
Morning			
Evening			
Saturday			
Morning			
Evening			
Sunday			
Morning			
Evening			

CHAPTER 4

Module 4: Behavioral Activation

Chapter Overview

This chapter focuses on behavioral activation for addressing depressive symptoms and isolation that occurs in the context of difficulty adjusting to changes in function from COVID-19. The exercises described in this part of the Therapist Guide are aimed at helping clients to re-engage with pleasurable activities abandoned due to COVID-19. Reintroducing meaningful activities that are rewarding and provide a sense of achievement can optimize the client's outlook and engagement in their life, despite potential limitations imposed by COVID-19. Figure 4.1 provides suggestions for modifications of activities based on physical/medical symptoms of COVID-19 and disability. Worksheet 4.1: Adapting Activities and Worksheet 4.2: Generating New Activities help the client problem-solve ways to engage in pleasurable activities in the context of the ongoing illness. Worksheet 4.3: Activity Schedule helps the client create a pleasant activities schedule.

Number of Sessions

The recommended number of sessions for this chapter is two or three, though ongoing pleasant activities scheduling can occur even as treatment progresses to additional chapters. Consider administering self-report symptom questionnaires (e.g., PHQ-9, GAD-7) at the beginning of the session to continue tracking symptoms of depression and anxiety.

Psychoeducation on Mood, Activities, and the Reward System

Humans have distinct brain structures that are responsible for processing rewarding sensations. These reward structures are thought to be underactive when people are depressed but can become "reactivated" when people engage in pleasurable activities and experience achievement (Pizzagali et al., 2009). Depression contributes to a reduced approach toward previously rewarding activities. For example, a depressed person who may have previously experienced reward from completing a difficult task or from social interactions may think, "I am worthless and no fun to be around." The combination of unpleasant thoughts and feelings can lead to amotivation to engage in work or social tasks, which perpetuates depressive symptoms.

Individuals experiencing persisting sequelae of COVID-19 may withdraw from typically rewarding experiences. Medical complications and ongoing physical symptoms can contribute to difficulties in carrying out mood-enhancing activities that brought pleasure and/or a sense of achievement prior to COVID-19. As such, individuals are robbed of the opportunity to be exposed to rewarding activities, which exacerbates mood difficulties.

Start by providing your client with the above psychoeducation on the association between mood and activity. Point out the bidirectional link between mood and activity—although low mood and depressive feelings tell us not to engage in activities, by reducing our engagement in pleasurable or achievement-oriented activities, mood can worsen further. The cycle becomes self-perpetuating. This cycle can be broken by starting to re-engage in activities that provide a sense of reward, meaning, pleasure, achievement, and/or mastery.

Behavioral Activation

One of the most widely supported cognitive behavioral techniques to reduce depression is behavioral activation (Lejuez et al., 2001). This technique aims to kick-start the experience of reward by helping clients generate and schedule plans to purposefully engage in activities that are pleasurable and/or promote achievement and mastery. As clients continue to engage in rewarding experiences, they simultaneously build experiences that can help them begin disproving negative thoughts by gathering real-life evidence.

Explain to the client that creating plans to carry out rewarding activities increases the chance that these activities occur. The goal in these sessions of therapy is to help clients understand the concept of behavioral activation, identify activities that are pleasurable or promote a sense of mastery/achievement, problem-solve barriers to engaging in activities, and schedule activities they could potentially enjoy. Once clients start engaging in activities that are rewarding, they are then encouraged to increase the frequency and intensity of rewarding behaviors over time. A weekly evaluation of "what went right" and assessment of barriers to carrying out plans can help clients troubleshoot and anticipate future hindrances to carrying out behavioral activation plans.

Adapting Activities for Persisting Sequelae of COVID-19

As part of this discussion, it will be important for you to acknowledge and validate that some activities that the client engaged in prior to COVID-19 may no longer be possible, at least in the exact same way as before, and at least at the current time. Persisting sequelae of COVID-19, such as mobility limitations, difficulties with sensation, shortness of breath, fatigue, and cognitive difficulties, can all pose very real barriers to engaging in activities. The client may be more reliant on others for transportation and accompaniment to activities. Help the client identify any potential barriers and explore to what extent the client feels limited by physical or medical barriers (versus their mood and depressive symptoms).

With your client in session, look at Figure 4.1, which appears in both the Client Workbook and the Therapist Guide. This figure focuses on illustrating ways to problem-solve activity engagement that is modified for those with physical/medical barriers and limitations. The goal here is not necessarily to fully replace the old activity with the new one. The examples of modifications given may not promote the same level

Previously enjoyed activity	Why did you enjoy it?	Barrier(s) preventing you from doing the activity now	Alternate activities that might help you connect with a similar sense of meaning, pleasure, or achievement
Weekly dinners with my extended family	Social connection, feeling like I was up to date on my family members' lives, enjoying good food	Can't drive anymore and don't have accessible transportation	Weekly video chats with my family. This will help me connect with them even though I can't enjoy the food. Try to plan monthly dinners and arrange for someone to drive me.
Working full-time as a healthcare worker	Camaraderie, helping other people, learning about new innovations in healthcare	Ongoing fatigue and brain fog prevent me from returning to work	Attend seminars so I keep learning about new innovations. Find a volunteer position for a few hours a week. Eventually try working part-time.
Participating in my church congregation	Sense of spirituality, teaching others, social connection	Ongoing need for supplemental oxygen makes it difficult to participate in a full church service	Participate in virtual church services, read religious scriptures, lead a virtual study group with congregation.
Long-distance running with my running team	Feeling strength and vitality, keeping in shape, motivating others on my team	Fatigue and mobility challenges mean I can only run short distances	Run short distances, add new physical activities to my workouts that my physical therapist suggested, text my running teammates so I can provide them with motivation
Dropping my kids off at school and picking them up in the afternoon	Contributing positively to my kids' development	My doctor told me I can't drive so my partner has to drive the kids to and from school	Help make and pack lunches for the kids. Take on a bigger role in helping my kids with their homework (my partner used to do more of this).

Figure 4.1.
Adapting Activities

of reward system activation in the same way as the prior activity, and there may still be a sense of loss for the client and frustration at what cannot be done. However, the goal is for the client to find reasonable approximations that may tap into the same values and meaning that the original activity did. Go over these examples with the client before turning to Worksheet 4.1: Adapting Activities, which is a blank version of an activity modification table. Worksheets can be found at the end of this chapter in both the Therapist Guide and Client Workbook or can be accessed by searching for this book's title on the Oxford Academic platform, at academic.oup.com.

Adapting Activities for Behavioral Activation

Collaboratively start to fill out Worksheet 4.1: Adapting Activities in your session. Have the client list activities that provide a sense of reward, meaning, pleasure, achievement, and/or mastery. Most of these will likely be activities that the client engaged in without too much difficulty prior to COVID-19. Next, ask the client *why* they enjoyed each activity—what was it about that activity that provided a sense of meaning or pleasure? Ask the client about any barriers associated with COVID-19 that have prevented them from engaging in the activity. Finally, turn to the fourth column to brainstorm alternate activities that could be attempted, which might tap into the same sense of meaning and purpose as the original activity. Note that this aspect of behavioral activation may be met with resistance, particularly if there are intense emotions such as anger or grief associated with the loss of the initial activity. There also may be an "all or nothing" approach to an activity, which leads the client to think, "If I can't do what I could do before, then I don't want to do anything at all." If this occurs, spend time exploring these thoughts and emotions with the client and validating the client's emotional experience and grief. Remind the client that withdrawing fully from activities typically has a negative impact on mood. Ask the client whether they would be willing to test a hypothesis and try out an alternate activity and track their mood to evaluate the impact of the activity on their mood.

Generating New Activities for Behavioral Activation

In addition to modifications to previous activities, Worksheet 4.2: Generating New Activities contains a section for novel activities that the client can try. Also included is a list of potential pleasurable activities if a client is having difficulty generating their own. Instead of modifying an old activity, the client may prefer to think of new activities. This is a perfectly valid approach, if the same tenets are followed in that the client ensures the activity is pleasurable and/or promotes achievement and mastery.

Encourage clients to revisit the list and add activities as they can over time. The following questions can help when probing for new activities:

"What are the things in life that give you meaning, purpose, and vitality—and what activities might help you connect with those feelings? What personal strengths do you have and what activities might help you demonstrate those strengths? If in the midst of this painful illness of COVID-19 there are strengths or qualities that you could develop and help you grow, what might they be—and what activities might help you achieve that? If in the future you looked back on this time, what would you like to say about the way you managed it?"

Therapist Note

Clients with limited resources may be more limited in the types of activities they can engage in. Individuals whose ability to work has been compromised by COVID-19-related sequelae may be facing financial challenges and may require support in brainstorming activities that are less financially dependent but that also provide meaning and pleasure. Clients who have very little income, are homebound, or who work long hours might also feel like they have little ability to do anything different with their time. In these cases, it is important that you work as creatively as possible to generate enjoyable and/or important activities within the client's limitations.

Activity Scheduling

Next, turn to Worksheet 4.3: Activity Schedule to collaborate with the client to create a pleasant activity schedule for the upcoming week, in session. Ask clients in session to choose two activities that they can complete each day. Activities should be chosen based on their potential to elicit pleasure or enhance the client's sense of achievement or increase social connectedness. Ask the client to enter the activities on Worksheet

4.3. Having a dedicated time and day to engage in activities makes it more likely for that activity to occur.

At-Home Practice

Review with your client the importance of at-home practice. For this week's homework, ask the client to implement the daily activity log created in session. Further, clients are asked to rate their sense of pleasure and sense of achievement after they have completed each activity. Provide clients with additional copies of the worksheet so they can continue to complete it weekly throughout the course of treatment as a means of intentionally engaging with positive emotions and increasing self-efficacy and mastery over their emotional experience during recovery.

Troubleshooting Barriers in Subsequent Sessions

Reviewing the completed activity schedule for the week at the beginning of each session helps to highlight the importance of behavior practice and mood tracking. If the client did not engage in the activities as planned, troubleshoot barriers to completion with the client, while continuing to reinforce the importance of out-of-session practice to positive treatment outcome. Incomplete homework should be worked on in part in session, but assignments in their entirety cannot be completed in session as the nature of the exercise for behavioral activation requires that clients devote time outside of session to engaging with their environment.

To probe for barriers, you might say to the client:

"What are some barriers you have noticed to completing activities? If you felt overwhelmed, were the barriers related to not having a specific time set? Not having the tools you needed at the right time (e.g., setting a time to read but spending time picking a book rather than having a book selected in order to begin reading)? Starting to re-engage in activities may seem like a lot of work, and if it feels too challenging to get started, we can re-evaluate the activities and break them down into smaller, more manageable bits. If tracking your pleasure ratings was the problem, let's

think about easier ways to do this (e.g., can you keep notes on your phone or email your ratings to yourself if you cannot find your paper calendar)?"

Sometimes it is tempting for clients to select very difficult activities that they were able to accomplish prior to their illness but that are now more challenging due to changes in mood and physical functioning. For example, going to work for a full day or taking a walk to their local grocery store may be things they were able to easily accomplish prior to their illness. Taking on activities that are not in line with their current level of functioning may backfire and contribute to demoralization. Work with clients to adjust to new functioning as they build manageable stepping stones toward improvement in mood and physical functioning while maintaining hope. Prioritize smaller goals to allow clients to build traction and momentum in engaging in activities and increasing rewarding experiences while enhancing motivation to take on larger challenges down the road.

Worksheet 4.1
Adapting Activities

Think of activities you previously enjoyed and write down what it was about those activities that gave you a sense of meaning, purpose, or enjoyment.

Previously enjoyed activity	Why did you enjoy it?	Barrier(s) preventing you from doing the activity now	Alternate activities that might help you connect with a similar sense of meaning, pleasure, or achievement

Worksheet 4.2
Generating New Activities

Think of new activities within the areas of work, leisure, physical activity, personal growth, and relationships. What new activities could you engage in that might give you a sense of meaning, purpose, enjoyment, or growth? Are there activities you could engage in that might help you demonstrate areas or strength (or develop new strengths)?

List of New Activities

Below is a list of activities that some people find pleasurable. See if you might be interested in trying any of these activities if you're having trouble generating activities on your own:

- Drink aromatic tea
- Hold your pet (if you have one)
- Call a friend

- Play cards
- Spend time in nature
- Text a friend

- Listen to music
- Cook a meal you enjoy
- Video chat with a friend

- Watch a new series on TV
- Eat a meal you enjoy
- Play a video game

- Dance, or tap your fingers to make a rhythm
- Write a letter to someone you care about
- Take a warm shower or bath

- Go to a religious service or listen to a recorded one
- Play an instrument or listen to a song
- Listen to a podcast

- Read a book
- Sit outside on a sunny day
- Use your phone to take pictures

- Listen to an audiobook
- Go to a neighborhood café or restaurant
- Make a list of things you're grateful for

Worksheet 4.3
Activity Schedule

Day/time	Activity to try (see Worksheets 4.1 and 4.2)	Pleasure after completing *Rate from 0 (no pleasure) to 10 (maximal pleasure)*	Sense of achievement after completing *Rate from 0 (feel no achievement) to 10 (feel maximal achievement)*
Monday Activity 1_____am/pm Activity 2_____am/pm	_____ _____	_____ _____	_____ _____
Tuesday Activity 1_____am/pm Activity 2_____am/pm	_____ _____	_____ _____	_____ _____
Wednesday Activity 1_____am/pm Activity 2_____am/pm	_____ _____	_____ _____	_____ _____
Thursday Activity 1_____am/pm Activity 2_____am/pm	_____ _____	_____ _____	_____ _____
Friday Activity 1_____am/pm Activity 2_____am/pm	_____ _____	_____ _____	_____ _____
Saturday Activity 1_____am/pm Activity 2_____am/pm	_____ _____	_____ _____	_____ _____
Sunday Activity 1_____am/pm Activity 2_____am/pm	_____ _____	_____ _____	_____ _____

CHAPTER 5

Module 5: Mindfulness

Chapter Overview

In this chapter, clients are introduced to mindfulness practice. The chapter includes psychoeducation, an experiential mindfulness exercise, and assignment of daily practice of mindfulness for at-home practice between sessions. The chapter contains Worksheet 5.1: Mindfulness for psychoeducation and for clients to log mindfulness practice.

Number of Sessions

We recommend spending at least one and up to three sessions on this chapter. The need for additional mindfulness sessions can be guided by case conceptualization and the client's presentation. For example, clients newer to psychotherapy and mindfulness practice may benefit from spending two or three sessions on this module of skills and additional mindfulness exercises. We also encourage you to create a plan with your clients for ongoing practice of mindfulness, even after moving on to later chapters within this program. Consider administering self-report symptom questionnaires (e.g., PHQ-9, GAD-7) at the beginning of the session to continue tracking symptoms of depression and anxiety.

Therapeutic Content

Information on Mindfulness for Therapists

Mindfulness is a term that has become increasingly popular among the public, as well as with mental health practitioners. While we acknowledge that practitioners have used varying definitions and conceptualizations of mindfulness over the years, we define mindfulness here and throughout this chapter as "paying attention in a particular way: on purpose, in the present moment, and non-judgmentally," a commonly cited definition proposed by Kabat-Zinn (2003). We present this definition to clients and walk them through a series of mindfulness practices to guide them in purposefully attending to the present moment, including their internal and external environments, while encouraging them to notice and let go of judgments about their experiences. While mindfulness meditation is one form of mindfulness practice, we want to clarify here that mindfulness practices are not highlighted as the sole form of meditative practices in this chapter. Other approaches may be useful as well. We have found clients with COVID-19 to specifically benefit from mindfulness in our work (Jaywant et al., 2021b, 2022).

Present Focus on Internal and External Stimuli

We present the practice of mindfulness as practicing non-evaluative attention to the "here and now." Paying attention to the present moment can be difficult, especially for clients who engage in worry or other unhelpful thoughts. Within the practice of mindfulness, the technique of observing a particular stimulus (such as an item in the external environment), noticing when one's attention inevitably drifts from that stimulus, acknowledging this without judgment, and returning one's attention to the stimulus of focus can help clients return to the present moment.

Over time the practice of returning attention to the "here and now" can help clients who are experiencing ongoing effects of COVID-19 to regain a sense of control over ruminative or unpleasant thoughts of past events or future worries that keep clients them in the uncertainty of the future (Desrosiers et al., 2013). Clients with ongoing COVID-19 symptoms experience frequent worries rooted in uncertainty about the future, including fears of worsening or indefinite physical and cognitive limitations (Moradi et al., 2020). Others report ongoing unhelpful preoccupation with past physical functioning and compare themselves to current physical limitations in an unhelpful or counterproductive manner. Clients might also experience ruminating thoughts surrounding the past and previous actions they engaged in, such as attending an event that led to them contracting COVID-19, or inadvertently exposing another person to COVID-19. Teaching clients to attend to the present moment purposefully and nonjudgmentally can provide relief from both distressing thoughts and feelings. Mindful awareness of one's experience can also play a role in meaningfully engaging with this treatment program—for example, by making clients more aware of their emotions, thoughts, and behaviors in the current moment.

Psychoeducation on Mindfulness

Case Vignette 5.1 illustrates how mindfulness can be introduced and discussed. Note how the therapist defines the concept and discusses its importance within this treatment program. Also explored is the client's existing understanding of mindfulness and any mindfulness or meditation practice conducted in the past.

Case Vignette 5.1

THERAPIST: *For today's session, we're going to be talking about and practicing mindfulness, and learning why mindfulness is an important skill to practice in this treatment program. I realize a lot of people have heard the term mindfulness before; have you?*

CLIENT: *Yeah, I've heard about it from friends and on social media.*

THERAPIST: *Absolutely, it's a concept that's gotten popular over the years. What do you think mindfulness is?*

CLIENT: *I don't know, really—it's like meditation, right? Like clearing your mind and relaxing? I feel like that all has sounded so "new age" and for hippies, and not really for me. I also feel like it's impossible for me to clear my head!*

THERAPIST: *Mindfulness has been spoken about a lot, especially these days, and I understand how the things you've heard about it or the people you've heard discussing meditation have made you feel like it's not for you. I also completely get that "clearing your mind" seems impossible for you to do! But did you know that mindfulness does not have to be practiced as a meditation, and that mindfulness can look like a lot of different things? And that it doesn't mean emptying your mind?*

CLIENT: *Really? What do you mean?*

THERAPIST: *Mindfulness is really defined as paying attention, on purpose, in the present moment, nonjudgmentally. So really, any time we are practicing paying attention to and noticing what's happening in the present moment, noticing what's happening inside and outside of ourselves, while letting go of judgments that inevitably will come up, we are practicing mindfulness. So we can practice mindfulness while meditating. But we can also practice mindfulness when trying to focus our attention on our breath or a sight or sound outside of our body and keep bringing our focus back to that anytime it wanders. We can also practice noticing our thoughts, emotions, and body sensations, while doing a lot of other things, like listening to music, taking a shower or bath, or even eating something.*

CLIENT: *OK, that makes sense, and sounds a lot easier than just trying to clear my head.*

THERAPIST: *Absolutely, anyone can practice mindfulness, and research shows that the more we practice, the easier it is to focus our attention on the present moment, because as people, we have a tendency for our minds to drift either to the past or the future. Have you ever noticed that?*

CLIENT: *Definitely! I have a bad habit of thinking a lot about the past and mistakes I've made. Or getting lost in how things used to be before I got COVID. I think I also live in the future a lot. I keep worrying about things I might not be able to do anymore, like running, because my breathing hasn't been the same since getting COVID. I try to not worry too much about the future but it's hard.*

THERAPIST: *I can imagine. And that's why mindfulness can be helpful, by keeping you more focused on the present. It takes practice. I'm wondering, have you been feeling upset or down and not sure why?*

CLIENT: *Definitely. I mean, I've been really depressed and anxious since getting COVID, since so much has changed since I caught it. And sometimes I feel OK, sometimes I feel absolutely depressed, and I don't always know why.*

THERAPIST: *That's very common. Mindfulness can help us better understand what's running though our minds, or what we are reacting to when we are feeling upset. And mindfulness can give us information about how to help ourselves. As "new age" as mindfulness sounds sometimes, there's decades of research showing how mindfulness practice can help improve our overall moods and functioning.*

CLIENT: *That sounds like it could be helpful.*

THERAPIST: *Definitely, and along the way we'll also practice noticing and letting go of judgments. We all have them. Ever notice that judgments can make you feel worse? Like judging yourself as incompetent, or other people are uncaring about you or selfish?*

CLIENT: *Yeah, I judge myself for not being able to do the things I used to do before COVID. I also judge myself for not being able to shake myself out of this funk.*

THERAPIST: *That sounds hard. With mindfulness practice, we also practice describing our-selves and situations in terms of facts, as opposed to unhelpful judgments.*

CLIENT: *That sounds challenging, but I'd be open to trying it.*

THERAPIST: *Fantastic. If it's OK with you, I'd like to lead us through a mindfulness practice in our work together, and you'll also be working on this for homework between our sessions. Sound good?*

Mindfulness Practice—Observing Emotions, Thoughts, and Bodily Sensations

Use the following Mindfulness Exercise and Case Vignette 5.2 to introduce the client to their first mindfulness practice in session. You will be orienting them to an "open awareness practice" to begin, which we find particularly useful to start with when working with clients newer to mindfulness practice. Keep in mind that observing emotions, thoughts, and bodily sensations may be done while engaging in any behavior. It can be helpful, however, to provide an anchor (such as listening to a piece of music) for clients newer to mindfulness practice to observe emotions, thoughts, and bodily sensations surrounding a particular stimulus.

Ask the client to maintain an upright sitting posture, either on a chair or on the floor, and attempt to maintain focus on a particular stimulus for a period of time. To begin mindfulness practice, we advise a practice of approximately 3 minutes in duration, followed by some time noting and describing observations that arose during that time.

Mindfulness Exercise

Case Vignette 5.2: Script for Mindfulness Practice: Observing Emotions, Thoughts, and Bodily Sensations

THERAPIST: *I'd like us to begin our mindfulness practice. Remember, the goal of our mind-fulness practice today will be to simply observe and notice. We will practice purposefully observing our internal experience during the next few minutes, while trying to let go of any judgments or unhelpful interpretations about our experience. The goal will be to notice our thoughts, emotions, bodily sensations, urges, or any memories, and then afterwards we can share what we both noticed with each other. How does that sound?*

CLIENT: *It sounds OK. What will we be observing?*

THERAPIST: *That's a great question, because as you can probably remember, we can observe our internal experiences of doing just about anything! However, for today, in order to make this easier, I'm going to ask you to notice anything that comes up for you while I play a song. It might be a song that's familiar to you, and if so, you might notice a memory and certain emotions come up for you while you listen to it again. It might also be a song that you've never heard before, and you'll want to notice with curiosity any thoughts, emotions, or urges that come up for you. And as always, with any mindfulness practice, we might simply notice our mind wandering all over the place, or an emotion that doesn't feel pleasant or comfortable! But that's OK, that's all part of the goal of mindfulness, which is to notice.*

CLIENT: *OK, got it.*

THERAPIST: *OK, so I'll begin playing a song shortly. While I play this, I invite you to keep your eyes closed to focus more fully on your internal experience than anything in your external environment. However, if that's too uncomfortable for you, you can instead choose to rest your gaze on some area where you can minimize distractions.*

[THERAPIST: Begins to play 3-minute piece of music.]

Selecting a stimulus to observe that, for most people, is particularly emotionally evocative can aid clients who are newer to mindfulness practice in observing elements of their internal experience. Therefore, we recommend that you choose a piece of music to play for mindfulness practice that is likely to be emotionally evocative or evoke particular memories for the client (Barlow et al., 2017). For example, you might select a song that was popular around the time your client was an adolescent or an early adult, such as a theme song from a popular show or movie or a slower song that might evoke sadness or contemplation. Alternately, you might consider songs that are upbeat and evoke urges to dance in most people. You might ask the client to share some of their favorite movies, television shows, or musical artists growing up to help in the selection of a song, and then repeat this mindfulness practice with a song of the client's choice.

Also, keep in mind that after listening to the piece of music mindfully, your client may have a hard time articulating observations of their mindfulness practice initially, and may benefit from modeling from you in order to do so. For example, you may share any thoughts or emotions, particular memories that arose, urges to dance and move, or distractions that you yourself noticed during the song. This sharing tends to aid the client in recalling any similar or disparate experiences and to normalize the experience of distraction and redirection of attention during mindfulness. Following completion of the song, debrief by exploring the client's experience with the practice using the script in Case Vignette 5.3.

Case Vignette 5.3: Script for Debriefing Experience of the Mindfulness Practice

---

THERAPIST: *OK, you can open your eyes if they were closed, or refocus on me if you kept them open. Now tell me, what are some things that you noticed when listening to this song?*

CLIENT: *Well, I noticed thinking of a movie that this was a soundtrack for when I was younger, so I found myself thinking about that movie for a while and losing focus on the song.*

THERAPIST: *That makes sense!*

CLIENT: *Yeah. And about halfway through the song I started to think about the lyrics and thinking about dancing to it. And I started to think that I'm probably not going to be able to dance for a while, maybe ever again, since I keep getting short of breath, and I started to feel sad.*

THERAPIST: *I hear you, and you did a fantastic job noticing all of that. Thank you for sharing with me what you noticed. And it's really important that you were able to observe those memories, thoughts, and even that feeling of sadness. Oftentimes people think that mindfulness is all about relaxation, or clearing one's mind, but noticing anything that's coming up in the present is important, even if it's hard or uncomfortable.*

CLIENT: *Why's that? I prefer not to notice those kinds of thoughts, as that's when I start to get down.*

THERAPIST: *I completely understand that. And if it were just so easy to push away sad thoughts and feelings, I'm sure you would have done so already. But really, all of those feelings are important and give important information—remember how we talked about that?*

CLIENT: *Yes* [recalling work from Chapter 3: Identifying and Understanding Your Emotions After COVID-19].

THERAPIST: *And even those thoughts are important, too. Remember how we talked about noticing unhelpful thoughts and how that will be part of our program, too? It all starts with catching the thoughts running through your head and noticing how they make you feel. And we go from there. We're going to have more opportunity to practice noticing our thoughts, though, with more practice.*

Following the first mindfulness practice, it is important to reinforce that the goal of mindfulness is not necessarily relaxation, nor is it to involve a meditative practice of clearing one's mind. Clients are being mindful anytime they are observing what is arising in the present, even when it's uncomfortable; when they are noticing or verbalizing what they are experiencing; and when they're letting go of unhelpful evaluations of the present moment.

At-Home Practice

Review with your client the importance of at-home practice. For homework, assign Worksheet 5.1: Mindfulness. This worksheet can be found at the end of this chapter in both the Therapist Guide and Client Workbook or can be accessed by searching for this book's title on the Oxford Academic platform, at academic.oup.com. For this at-home practice assignment, ask clients to practice mindful observing for 3 minutes each day. The client will use the worksheet to log their experience and will complete it independently at home. However, when assigning the worksheet, it can be helpful to briefly brainstorm and plan which activities in the following week the client wants to practice being mindful. This can include, for example, eating a piece of fruit and paying mindful attention to the smell, taste, and texture of the fruit; or taking a bath and noticing the feeling of water against the skin. The client will practice observing and noting the thoughts, emotions, and bodily sensations that arise.

Also when assigning Worksheet 5.1, it is helpful to discuss any anticipated barriers, and help the client to plan ahead for how to circumvent them. Troubleshooting potential barriers might involve the client setting daily reminders on their mobile device, and/or arranging to minimize distractions during the selected period of time that will be dedicated to the practice of mindfulness skills.

Cultural Considerations

Variations in mindfulness practice can be seen across cultures (Tadlock-Marlo, 2011). While mindfulness meditation has its roots in Buddhism, individuals across spiritual, ethnic, and cultural groups have the capability of using mindfulness to cultivate present-moment awareness (Gunaratana, 2011). When working with clients from non-Western cultural backgrounds, you can encourage mindfulness practice while engaging in other culturally relevant activities. You can instruct clients to engage in such activities like dancing, cooking, and prayer as a mindfulness practice, attending to those activities without distraction.

At the same time, some clients may report that practicing mindfulness is incongruent with their religious beliefs or spiritual traditions. If this is the case, remind clients that they have a choice to not engage in mindfulness practices as described in this chapter as doing so may violate their values or be perceived as disrespectful. However, be sure to explore your client's definition of mindfulness, as simply attending to what is happening in the present moment without judgment typically does not violate the tenets of many religious and spiritual practices.

Mobile Apps

Several mobile apps currently exist that can help clients in their mindfulness practices outside of session (Mani et al., 2015). The apps range in price, and offer various guided meditations and breathing practices that can supplement clients' practice of mindfulness as part of this treatment program. Some mindfulness mobile apps may be effective (Flett et al., 2019), and as such you may consider encouraging clients to use them to augment their between-session mindfulness practice.

Once the client has demonstrated increased awareness of their internal experiences and has developed a plan for continued practice, you may move on to further chapters within this program.

Worksheet 5.1
Mindfulness

"Paying attention, on purpose, to the present"

- Noticing: becoming fully aware of our thoughts, emotions, physical sensations, and environment in the present moment
- Bringing curiosity, openness, and interest to our experience
- Being nonjudgmental toward our experience. Notice the urge to judge or react to our experience and just observe our thoughts and emotions like they were clouds in the sky.

Benefits of Mindfulness

- Promoting present-moment focus. Persistent symptoms of COVID-19 can lead us to feel down on ourselves over past mistakes, long for the life that used to be, and worry for the future. By keeping our awareness on the present, we can decrease symptoms of anxiety and depression.
- Mindfulness teaches us how to focus, expand, or redirect our attention. It helps us notice where our attention is, when it has wandered, and bring it back to the present.
- When we mindfully observe painful thoughts and emotions, we gain some distance from them and feel less "stuck" in them. Mindfulness can help us be more compassionate toward ourselves, our emotions, and our experiences.

How to Practice

- Mindfulness can be practiced anytime, anywhere.
- It can be helpful to dedicate a few minutes every day for mindfulness practice.
- Try to keep your practice as consistent as possible across days. This will help it become more routine and automatic.

Choose an activity to engage in mindfully for 3 minutes each day. Tasks can include eating, listening to music, walking, or breathing. During the 3 minutes of your practice, intentionally observe your inner experience while engaging in the task by noticing the thoughts, emotions, memories, and bodily sensations that arise. Alternatively, use a guided recording.

Day	Activity to Practice Mindfulness	Noteworthy Observations
Monday		
Tuesday		
Wednesday		
Thursday		
Friday		
Saturday		
Sunday		

CHAPTER 6

Module 6: Relaxation Skills

Chapter Overview

This chapter is intended to provide background and training in relaxation skills to help clients manage acute emotional distress. Topics covered include psychoeducation on the acute stress response and the physiological basis of and mechanisms behind relaxation strategies. The client is also introduced to specific relaxation exercises and barriers to participation, as well as special considerations. Box 6.1 and Box 6.2 include scripts for relaxation exercises. The chapter contains Worksheets 6.1: Self-Soothing Skills, 6.2: Soothing Self-Statements, 6.3: Distraction Skills, 6.4: Relaxation Practice Record, and 6.5: My Relaxation Plan.

Number of Sessions

The recommended number of sessions is two or three, with additional sessions necessary for clients who present with acute emotional distress and/or require additional practice of relaxation skills. Consider administering self-report symptom questionnaires (e.g., PHQ-9, GAD-7) at the beginning of the session to continue tracking symptoms of depression and anxiety.

Therapeutic Content

Overview of the Acute Stress Response

Clients may be unfamiliar with the fight-or-flight response. Psychoeducation on the fight-or-flight response can help clients recovering from COVID-19 understand why certain physiological sensations arise and continue to be present in moments of acute distress (e.g., why their body reacts and feels the way it does).

Explain to the client that stress is something we all experience at one time or another. Acute stress is immediate stress that occurs in everyday life and is often accompanied by physical sensations. The fight-or-flight response (also known as hyperarousal or the acute stress response) is a physiological response to a stimulus that is perceived as stressful or frightening. The acute stress response begins in the brain (amygdala), which then activates the autonomic nervous system. The autonomic nervous system controls involuntary or automatic (not consciously directed) bodily functions like breathing, heart rate, blood pressure, and digestive processes. The autonomic nervous system is divided into the sympathetic and parasympathetic nervous systems. The *sympathetic nervous system* directs the body's fight-or-flight response. It prepares the body to respond to a perceived threat, danger, or stressor. It is our body's "emergency alarm system" and causes a number of physical changes that keep our body "revved up" or on high alert. The *parasympathetic nervous system* prompts the "rest and digest" response—it helps to keep us relaxed and calms the body down after a stressful event.

In the context of COVID-19, triggers for the fight-or-flight response may include physiological sensations like shortness of breath, attending medical visits, or going to locations perceived to have a high rate of re-infection risk (e.g., an indoor concert, a busy grocery store). Explaining to clients the automatic or involuntary nature of the acute stress response can be validating for those who view it as a sign that they are "losing control" or believe it is their "fault" they are experiencing these sensations.

Symptoms of the Fight-or-Flight Response

When faced with a situation that causes significant anxiety, fear, or discomfort, the body responds with sudden, involuntary symptoms that are regulated by the sympathetic nervous system. These include faster heart rate, increased blood pressure, faster or more shallow breathing, pale or flushed skin, increased sharpness in hearing and vision, pupil dilation, and feeling tense or on edge. Other common symptoms associated with acute distress include muscle tension (tensing of the jaw, fists, shoulders, back, etc.), stomach discomfort, and chest tightness. Clients may also notice a lack of clarity of thought—racing, spiraling thoughts and difficulties problem-solving or focusing on the task at hand. Notably, these symptoms can overlap with those frequently experienced post-COVID-19 and can therefore have a reinforcing or reciprocal effect.

Review these symptoms with your client and elicit a recent moment of acute distress. For example:

- What was the situation?
- What was going through their mind?
- How were they feeling?
- Did they notice physiological sensations in their body?
- Have they reacted like this before?

It's important to emphasize to the client that the acute stress response is reflexive. It's a cascade of events that happens quite quickly and automatically, almost instantaneously after the stressor or danger is perceived. This is why we are able to slam on the breaks to avoid a car accident, even before we've had a chance to fully process what's happening.

Evolution of the Fight-or-Flight Response: Fear Without Danger

The client is likely to have some background on the adaptiveness of the fight-or-flight response in the setting of fear (Chapter 3). It is helpful to expand on it here for the purpose of teaching relaxation skills. Providing a brief background on the origin and role of the fight-or-flight response can help to normalize and destigmatize the symptoms. It's important to discuss how the stress response has evolved and distinguish when it is helpful (immediate danger) and when it is not.

The fight-or-flight response is an evolutionary defense mechanism that developed as a means of physical survival. Our very early ancestors were contending with true danger around every corner, and the fight-or-flight response evolved to activate human beings to respond quickly to threat. In today's world, immediate life-threatening situations are less common. The fight-or-flight response continues to be a helpful response in moments of true physical danger—for instance, jumping out of the way of an oncoming car. The fight-or-flight response can also be triggered by non–life-threatening experiences like acute stress. Some individuals experience an overactive stress response—when the body

101

becomes hypersensitive to stressors that are not life-threatening, like work pressure, traffic jams, and attending medical visits or rehabilitation sessions. In these individuals, the acute stress response can be triggered too frequently or at inappropriate times, due to a range of stressors. When the stress response is activated, our body is reacting "as if" we are in acute physical danger—when that is not actually the case. This can cause the non–life-threatening situation to *feel* just as dire as one that is truly dangerous. Thus, while adaptive in a life-threatening situation, experiencing fight-or-flight symptoms when driving, grocery shopping, or sitting in a meeting at work can be disruptive and frightening.

Therapist Note

Clients may assign meaning to the fight-or-flight symptoms such as "I'm having a heart attack," "There's something wrong with me/my body," or "I'm going to die." Some clients may try to escape situations as soon as they begin to notice the symptoms, instinctively believing they are dangerous, leading to maladaptive avoidance of activities. Explore this with the client. Are there specific triggers they notice or activities they avoid? Avoidance is common among those with an overactive or heightened stress response and only serves to reinforce the association of fear with the stimuli.

A key point is that certain medical conditions—such as COVID-19—and the accompanying experience with medical treatment can make clients more vulnerable to an overactive or sensitized stress response. This is illustrated in Case Vignette 6.1. For instance, clients with a pre-existing anxiety disorder are more likely to feel worried or fearful of non-threatening stressors, which can result in hyperarousal and an exaggerated response to daily activities or sources of distress (e.g., riding the bus, sitting in traffic). Severe acute medical illness or trauma, as many of our clients may have experienced prior to or during COVID-19 illness, can also lead to an exaggerated stress response. It will be helpful to evaluate the circumstances of the client's COVID-19 infection and treatment and any changes they've noticed in their response to stressors following COVID-19. Evidence also suggests that stressful events in childhood can lead to long-term abnormalities of the stress response system (Heim et al., 2008). Evaluation of early life adversity can help you inform conceptualization and application of relaxation strategies.

Case Vignette 6.1

Christine tested positive for COVID-19. She began to notice some fatigue and shortness of breath, and she went to the walk-in clinic for an evaluation. She anticipated this would be a brief and informative evaluation and that she'd be home in time to fix dinner for her wife and daughter before they returned home. At the clinic, Christine was given supplemental oxygen, and 24 hours later she was hospitalized, intubated, and placed on a mechanical ventilator. The ventilator was removed 3 weeks later, and she woke up with a foggy memory of the events leading up to her hospitalization. Given the unexpected nature of these medical events and the subsequent complications she faced, Christine began to fear even routine medical follow-ups with her providers, believing even standard appointments could lead to another prolonged hospitalization. Routine visits and reminder calls would trigger an acute stress response. Her heart would race and her face would flush when she started getting ready for appointments, which exacerbated her fear and discomfort. She began avoiding appointment reminders and canceling or rescheduling upcoming visits. In Christine's case, she is experiencing a generalized fear response to a previously neutral situation, getting routine medical care, as her body has erroneously assigned life-threatening significance to it given her unexpected and prolonged hospitalization. In fact, this association is leading Christine to avoid medical recommendations, and this could have serious health implications.

Background and Psychoeducation on the Relaxation Response

Provide the following psychoeducation to your client. Relaxation strategies are behavioral approaches to counteract the acute stress response. Relaxation strategies are designed to decrease physiological arousal and alleviate symptoms of acute stress. Relaxation strategies activate the parasympathetic nervous system, which acts like a brake pedal or the body's "off switch" to the fight-or-flight response (Esch et al., 2003; Hoffman et al., 1982). We can do this, for example, by redirecting our attention to the present moment, taking slower, deeper breaths, and releasing tension we may be holding in our body. Along with calming the body, many of these skills also help to calm the mind (Klainin-Yobas et al., 2015; Manzoni et al., 2008). During periods of heightened anxiety and distress, we can use these strategies to reduce physiological arousal and the emotional intensity of the moment.

After providing psychoeducation, ask the client whether they currently have any specific strategies they use to cope with moments of acute distress. Are they effective? Do they help in the short term but hurt in the long term (e.g., reaching for an alcoholic beverage)? Encourage any adaptive strategies the client currently uses. If the client identifies maladaptive or unhelpful strategies, discuss how the skills presented in this chapter are advantageous, and how they may be used to replace maladaptive or less productive alternatives. When discussing the specific benefits of relaxation, ask the client to identify benefits that are most important or meaningful to them.

Deciding When Relaxation Strategies Are Helpful

Relaxation skills should be used in moments of acute hyperarousal and emotional distress. The central goal is to help clients endure acute distress by reducing the intensity of the moment and reaching a state that allows other therapeutic strategies (mindfulness, cognitive restructuring) to work. Overuse of relaxation can get in the way of problem-solving and meaningful change and may counterproductively lead to emotional and behavioral avoidance. The factors listed below, adapted from the *DBT Skills Training Manual* (Linehan, 2014), outline the specific symptoms and circumstances that warrant the use of relaxation strategies.

- The client feels they are in an acute emotional crisis. They are having difficulty processing information effectively, are feeling emotionally overwhelmed, are caught up in racing thoughts they cannot contain, or notice physiological symptoms of the acute stress response.
- The level of distress and arousal is so high that the use of other skills is not feasible.
- The client has the urge to act impulsively or make a snap decision without thinking it through.

- An important task needs to be done, but they're too overwhelmed to problem-solve or think through what to do.
- When the client anticipates a stressful event or situation likely to trigger the acute stress response (e.g., returning to a hospital for the first time since their COVID-19-related hospitalization), relaxation can help to lower baseline physiological arousal prior to highly stressful situations and may help to weaken the acute stress response or enable use of other therapeutic strategies.

When Relaxation Strategies Are Unhelpful

Relaxation should not be used to avoid unwanted sensations and emotions. If clients try to control mild to moderate anxiety with relaxation, it does not allow them to fully experience their anxiety. Thus, misapplied relaxation can hinder clients from learning that they can tolerate their anxiety, and that discomfort does not mean danger. Explain to the client that relaxation should *not* be used the instant they begin to feel anxious or mild tension starts to build. Only when the intensity of the symptoms reaches a certain threshold (determined collaboratively with the client) should relaxation be used (see Case Vignette 6.2). Reducing arousal with relaxation allows the client to then engage in productive skill use. Following relaxation, it is important for the client to use a different therapeutic skill that's appropriate to the stressor or the symptoms.

Therapist Note

It can often help to identify a Subjective Units of Distress Scale (SUDS) severity/cut-off to initiate relaxation strategies. Over time, it may help to revise the symptom intensity threshold to signal the need for use of relaxation strategies. For example, at the start of treatment, the client and therapist determine that the client should use relaxation strategies when they reach a SUDS level of 7 out of 10 or greater. As treatment progresses and the client learns they can sit with discomfort, the intensity is increased so the client only applies relaxation skills at a SUDS level of 8 or higher.

Case Vignette 6.2

Erin just started a new job, and she received what she perceived as negative feedback from her boss. She has experienced cognitive difficulties post-COVID-19 and worries about her ability to perform at work. She has a new baby at home, and her husband is on leave from work to care for their baby. Finances have been a major concern and source of stress for their family in recent years. Erin quickly notices her telltale signs of acute distress (shallow breathing, racing heart, trembling, racing thoughts that feel out of control). She identifies her SUDS level as 8 out of 10. She steps into her office and engages in diaphragmatic breathing and pairs this with a self-soothing statement ("I can get through this") every time she exhales. She does this exercise for 5 minutes and then evaluates her physical symptoms and SUDS level. Now that she's reached a SUDS level of 6 out of 10, she begins to use cognitive reframing strategies to evaluate the evidence.

Relaxation Strategies

For in-session exercises, ask clients to rate their discomfort or distress (using a 0-to-10 SUDS or similar scale) before and after the exercise. Some clients, particularly those with prolonged hospitalizations, may have devices at home that monitor their vital signs (pulse oximeter, blood pressure monitor). To underscore the physiological benefits of relaxation, you may also ask the client to measure their heart rate or blood pressure prior to and after the exercise. Note that clients with ongoing respiratory difficulty and/or oxygen requirements may be reluctant to start with a breathing exercise, and thus imagery, progressive muscle relaxation, or self-soothing strategies may be a better starting point. Introducing strategies and giving the client a choice can be helpful here.

> **Therapist Note: Setting Expectations for Relaxation**
> *It is important for clients to maintain realistic expectations of these strategies so they don't abandon this set of skills because they believe they are ineffective. Set expectations in the beginning and emphasize the role*

of practice: "You may find that relaxation skills help you feel better. If that's the case, that's great. But if not, that doesn't mean the skills aren't working. Relaxation is not meant to take you from a place of extreme anxiety and worry to complete relaxation. It's very unlikely that you'll feel 100 percent or even 75 percent better. Instead, relaxation is meant to 'turn down the temperature' of those symptoms. Any decrease in the intensity of your symptoms (10 percent reduction in anxiety, less muscle tension) indicates effectiveness. In some cases, you may not even feel better than when you started the relaxation practice. However, it likely prevented you from feeling even worse. This is particularly the case when you first start practicing relaxation. Just like with learning any new skill, the techniques may feel awkward or unhelpful in the beginning. The effectiveness of relaxation improves with time and repetition, so with practice you'll find that you are able to become increasingly and deeply relaxed."

Skill 1: Diaphragmatic Breathing

Also known as abdominal breathing or belly breathing, diaphragmatic breathing allows the client to take deep, refreshing breaths and encourages full oxygen exchange. When we breath normally, we often breathe only into our upper chest, sucking our abdomen in slightly as we inhale. During diaphragmatic breathing, the client intentionally uses their diaphragm to take deep breaths, drawing air into the lower lungs, allowing them to use their lungs at greater capacity. To do diaphragmatic breathing, use this script:

"Make yourself comfortable. Rest your back in the chair with your feet on the floor. Place your hands at your sides or gently in your lap. Place one hand on your upper chest and the other on your belly, just below the ribcage. Breathe in deeply and slowly through your nose, toward your belly, so that your stomach moves out. Try to keep the hand on your chest still, while the one on your belly should rise as you take a slow, gentle inhale for several seconds. When breathing toward the belly, think about expanding your abdomen and widening the sides of your waist as you inhale.

"Purse your lips as if you are sipping through a straw. Exhale slowly through the lips for several seconds and feel the stomach gently contract. Make the exhale longer than the inhale. *As you breathe out, the hand*

on your belly should lower while the hand on your chest remains as still as possible. Through your nose, take another deep, slow inhale into the belly. Now gently and slowly, breathe out through your pursed lips. Repeat for at least 10 breath cycles."

Supportive prompts can be used during the practice, such as:

- *"Focus on the rhythm of your breathing."*
- *"Notice the sensation of the inhale, the coolness of the breath as it enters the nostrils."*
- *"If your mind wanders, that's OK. Just gently bring your thoughts back to your breath."*
- *"Notice the sensation of your belly rising and falling."*
- *"As you inhale, imagine breathing in feelings of calm and relaxation."*

Skill 2: Numbered Breathing

This strategy helps to slow the rate of breathing and focus the mind on the breath. It is simple and quick and can be done anywhere. The addition of a mental count can help to maintain focus on the breath. Instruct the client to count slowly; for example, a count of 4 should equal 4 seconds. To demonstrate numbered breathing, use this script:

"Take a slow, deep inhale through your nose for a count of 4. Hold your breath for a count of 7. Exhale slowly and completely through your mouth, making a whoosh sound, to a mental count of 8. Complete at least five breath cycles.

"If 4–7–8 feels too challenging to begin with, try shortening the breath cycles to 3–4–5 (in for 3, hold for 4, out for 5). Also feel free to exhale through your nose rather than your mouth, if that feels more comfortable for you."

Skill 3: Five-Finger Breathing

This is another strategy to help the client slow down and focus on the breath. The integration of tracing the hand helps with pacing the breath. It also helps to shift focus to the gentle sensation of touch along with deep breathing. To practice the five-finger breathing technique, use this script:

"Place one hand in front of you and spread your fingers apart. Use the pointer finger of the opposite hand to softly trace up the outside of the thumb as you take a deep, slow inhale. As you exhale, gently trace down the inside of the thumb. (Spend 4 to 5 seconds tracing upward on the inhale, and 4 to 5 seconds tracing downward on the exhale.) Repeat this for the pointer finger and the remaining fingers. Make sure to inhale as you trace up the finger, and exhale as you trace down."

"For each of the exercises above, try your best to keep your focus on your breath. Notice the rhythm of your breath, the cool sensation of the inhale through your nose, and the warmth of the exhale through your nose or mouth. Notice the sensation of your chest and belly, rising and falling as you breathe in and out. If your mind wanders, that's OK. It happens to everyone, even seasoned practitioners who have been doing it for many years. Each and every time you lose focus, mindfully bring your attention back to your breath."

Therapist Note: Why Breathing Works

For clients hesitant to engage in breathing-based exercises, it can help to provide additional psychoeducation on the process—that is, why breathing works. Explain that although breathing-based strategies may feel rather passive, they have established physiological benefits. We typically take 12 to 16 breaths per minute, and during acute stress breathing may become even faster and shallower. Engaging in deep breathing and associated exercises helps move us out of fight-or-flight mode by quieting sympathetic nervous system activity and activating the parasympathetic (rest-and-digest) response. This is achieved, in part, by stimulating the vagus nerve. The vagus nerve is a crucial cranial nerve that connects the brain to the body and plays a key role in facilitating communication between them. It helps the body switch back and forth between sympathetic and parasympathetic activity. In moments of acute distress, intentionally slowing down our breathing to 5 to 7 breaths a minute stimulates the vagus nerve, which communicates with the parasympathetic nervous system to produce a relaxation response. As a result, the body moves toward a state of physiological relaxation, where blood pressure, heart rate, temperature, and other biological processes return to normal.

Skill 4: Imagery

Developing a calming mental image can help the client create a relaxed state by pulling them away from stressful thoughts and sensations.
During this in-session exercise, the client imagines themselves in a
relaxing place, a place they associate with feelings of joy, warmth, and
restfulness—a place that they have been or would like to be that makes
them feel safe and calm. Imagery creates distance from the source of
distress and allows the client to instead shift their focus to a place of
peace and relaxation. Box 6.1: Beach Imagery Relaxation Exercise is an
example script that involves using the five senses to create a soothing
mental image to promote feelings of relaxation.

Box 6.1 Beach Imagery Relaxation Exercise

Start by making yourself comfortable. Lie down in a comfortable place with your head
supported. If you're seated in a chair, allow your arms to rest softly on your lap or at your
sides, and place your feet on the ground. Gently allow your eyes to close or remain open
with a soft gaze.

Bring your attention to your breath. Draw a deep breath in 2, 3, 4 . . . hold 2, 3 . . . and
exhale 2, 3, 4, 5. Breathe in again 2, 3, 4 . . . hold 2, 3 . . . and exhale 2, 3, 4, 5. Breathe
in again, slowly . . . pause for a moment . . . and breathe out.

Now, bring your attention to your body and scan your body for any tension you may be
holding. Continue to breathe in fully and exhale slowly, at your own pace. As you exhale,
release any tension you may be holding in your muscles, allowing your muscles to feel
loose, limp, and relaxed.

Now, as you continue breathing, begin to create a picture in your mind. Imagine you are
walking toward a quiet, secluded beach. It's early in the morning; the sun has just risen. The
temperature is comfortable, inviting, and warm. You breathe in the fresh, crisp ocean air.

As you reach the edge of the beach, you see the vibrant blue-green of the water and hear
the gentle waves up ahead. You walk further and feel the soft, smooth sand, warm against
your feet. A light breeze brushes against your cheek and shoulders. You can smell the salty
ocean spray. The waves glisten in the sun.

You walk toward the water, at a comfortable, slow pace. As you come closer, you hear the
waves washing up onto the shore—a comforting, predictable rhythm, flowing in and out.

Continue taking deep, gentle breaths. Breathe in fully and exhale slowly, at your own pace. Feel the tension flow out of your body as you admire the soothing scenery around you.

If your mind wanders, that's OK. Just gently bring your thoughts back to your breath and this place of peace and relaxation.

You step lightly into the water's edge, allowing the waves to wash over your feet and ankles. The sand is wet and firm beneath your feet. The water is a pleasant relaxing temperature, cool and comfortable. You feel the gentle pull of the waves as they flow in and out. The water is a clear blue, and you can see the white sand beneath it.

Picture yourself walking along the water's edge . . . free of worries . . . no stress . . . no responsibilities, feeling calm and relaxed. Feel the warmth of the sun on your skin, the soft sand at your feet, and the crisp, cool water on your toes and ankles. Breathe in the fresh ocean air. Fill your lungs completely. Gently and slowly exhale, releasing any tension as you breathe out.

To your right is a lush, tropical forest. Enjoy the rich combination of colors in the forest—the darkness of the bark on the trees, the deep greens of the leaves, and the vibrant hues of the tropical flowers. You feel a soft, gentle breeze on your skin. You notice the leaves sway delicately in the wind as a breeze blows through the forest. You hear birds and the soft, gentle rustling of the leaves.

As you imagine yourself in this place, continue to breathe in fully and exhale slowly, at your own pace.

Up ahead is a lounge chair and towel, set up just for you.

Imagine yourself walking toward the lounge chair, right at the shore of the coastline. You take a comfortable seat. You are fully supported in this moment, your feet grounded on the warm, soft sand and your body resting comfortably in the chair. Next to you is a fresh glass of ice water. As you pick it up, you feel the refreshing coolness of the glass on your fingertips and hear the delicate clink of the ice cubes. Imagine yourself taking a sip of the ice water, the refreshing feeling on your tongue, the coolness as you drink it. The sand is velvety soft and warm beneath your feet. You feel at peace, relaxed in this moment.

You can return to this place whenever you wish. It is always with you, safely tucked in your mind.

When you're ready, gradually shift your attention and awareness back to this room. Gently begin to open your eyes and become fully alert and refreshed.

Box 6.2 Your Imagery Relaxation Exercise

Start by making yourself comfortable. Bring your attention to your breath and take several slow, deep breaths. As you continue breathing, begin to create a picture in your mind. Imagine yourself seated or walking through a soothing environment of your choice.

See: What do you see? What catches your eye? What is in your line of sight? Try to imagine the specific details of the environment—the shapes, textures, colors, contours of your surroundings.

Hear: What sounds do you notice? Are there birds chirping, leaves flowing in the wind, the rhythm of the ocean waves?

Touch: What can you touch or feel (your feet on the soft grass, the warmth of the sand)? What sensations do you notice on your skin (a cool breeze on your cheek, the warmth of the sun)?

Smell: What does the air smell like—fresh, crisp? What other smells do you notice (e.g., pine trees, freshly cut grass, salty ocean air)?

Taste: Is there anything that you can taste (saltiness of the ocean air)? If not, picture yourself drinking a cool glass of ice water or lemonade for a warm location, or a soothing drink like herbal tea or cocoa for a cold location.

Spend 5 to 10 minutes taking gentle, deep breaths and imagining yourself in this place of peace and relaxation.

The client can also use their five senses to create a more personalized immersive experience and make the imagery even more effective. The instructions and script in Box 6.2: Your Imagery Relaxation Exercise can be used to try this out.

Distraction and Self-Soothing Techniques

Self-soothing and distraction can help to shift the client's focus away from the acute stressor and reset bodily systems during moments of acute distress. These practices can help achieve a more relaxed state by purposefully turning attention away from the acute stressor to things that feel pleasant and comforting. Worksheet 6.1: Self-Soothing Skills contains a comprehensive list of sensory-based self-soothing strategies.

Worksheets can be found at the end of this chapter in both the Therapist Guide and Client Workbook or can be accessed by searching for this book's title on the Oxford Academic platform, at academic.oup.com. Using the five senses can help the client to refocus on aspects of the physical world and anchor attention to the present moment. Evoking different sensations can create space from internal thoughts and redirect attention to something other than the emotional distress and its source. Review the list of sensory-based self-soothing strategies outlined in the worksheet. Ask clients to identify the methods they might be willing to try, and encourage them to offer their own methods.

Soothing Self-Statements

Self-soothing statements can also reduce acute distress and the intensity of the moment. These can serve as reminders to help the client ground themselves in the present moment and to prevent them from getting too wrapped up in the stressor or the intense emotions they are experiencing. Worksheet 6.2: Soothing Self-Statements can be done in session or assigned to the client as homework.

Distraction Strategies

Through distraction, the client can offset acute distress by redirecting their attention to enjoyable, productive, or meaningful activities. Be sure to distinguish distraction in moments of acute distress from maladaptive avoidance (e.g., of medical visits, physical therapy exercises). Direct the client to Worksheet 6.3: Distraction Skills. Ask the client to identify a few distracting skills they think might work for them and collaboratively develop a specific and concrete plan for using distracting activities under various circumstances.

At-Home Practice

Explain to the client that, like with learning anything new, practice is essential. Review the importance of out-of-session practice at home. Without practice, the strategies are difficult to engage when they're needed most. With practice, however, the skills will become more effective and more automatic and can be used anytime, anywhere, and with very little effort. Remind the client that relaxation enables the body to respond differently to stress. It reduces the impact of stressors and helps the client to recover and regain a sense of calm. Learning how to achieve this—by taking the time to learn these skills—is a worthwhile investment.

When beginning relaxation practice, clients should do the chosen exercise twice a day. Direct the client to Worksheet 6.4: Relaxation Practice Record, and assign this worksheet for homework. Remember, worksheets can be found at the end of this chapter in both the Therapist Guide and Client Workbook or can be accessed by searching for this book's title on the Oxford Academic platform, at academic.oup.com. Ask the client to use this form to rate their tension prior to and after the exercise and briefly record any changes in mood, thoughts, or physical sensations that they notice, even if subtle. Review the completed worksheet with the client at the start of each session. Practice at first should take place *during non-stressful moments* rather than during stressful situations. Practicing the skills outside of times of acute stress will make the strategies more effective in times of need.

Consider recording one of the above in-session practices or providing a guided audio to the client. This ensures that the client has access to the practice between sessions. Clients new to relaxation may find it difficult to do the practice independently, without any external guidance, but over time they will progress to practicing without the recording.

Create a Customized Relaxation Plan

In your next session, once the client has experience practicing a selected relaxation exercise or two independently, it is helpful to identify a selection of relaxation strategies that the client can draw upon at various times and in various circumstances. Some techniques may be more helpful than others, or some may be more effective in certain circumstances. After introducing various techniques to the client and following self-monitoring and practice (during and between sessions), collaboratively create a list of strategies with the client.

Introduce Worksheet 6.5: My Relaxation Plan in session and discuss with the client the strategies they've found to be most effective. Create a hierarchy of options (e.g., if numbered breathing doesn't work, try imagery). In addition, explore potential barriers to their use, and problem-solve ways to implement them. Identify preferences regarding strategy use in different situations and environments (e.g., some clients may be more comfortable than others using five-finger breathing in public).

Therapist Note: Mindfulness Versus Relaxation

Relaxation and mindfulness can sometimes have similar effects on our mood and mental state. Both can produce a sense of calm, and, like mindfulness, relaxation strategies often require a focus on the present moment. There are also some important differences. Mindfulness is a state of present-moment awareness, acceptance, and nonjudgment. While relaxation is often a byproduct of mindfulness, that is not the primary aim. Relaxation, in contrast, is a behavioral strategy to manage acute distress by calming the mind and modulating autonomic nervous system activity. Unlike relaxation, mindfulness focuses on accepting painful experiences and discomfort rather than changing, reducing, or avoiding them. Both approaches can be helpful for client well-being. Relaxation strategies can be integrated with, and used to complement, mindfulness techniques. They may also be differentially applied depending on the situation.

Addressing Barriers to Relaxation

▪ **"These strategies make me feel uncomfortable and anxious, not relaxed."** For many clients recovering from COVID-19, relaxation skills can lead to more anxiety initially, when they first begin to practice. Normalize this and explain that the body is very accustomed to responding to stress in one way, and teaching it to respond differently takes time and practice. It can even feel awkward, unnatural, or forced in the beginning. Assure the client that the anxiety response is common and short-lived. Emphasize that individuals who tend to have the most trouble with relaxation are also typically those who need it the most. For clients who feel particularly distressed or triggered by breathing exercises because of ongoing respiratory problems, we recommend focusing on non–breathing-related relaxation exercises such as imagery and distraction.

- **"I've tried breathing and relaxation before. It doesn't work for me."** Some clients may have already tried various mobile apps or resources and then discontinued them after not noticing any benefit. Normalize this and explain that many people do not notice significant benefit at first. Like with learning any new skill, the more they practice the easier and more effective it becomes. In addition, various judgments and beliefs ("I'm not doing this right") can get in the way. Explore these and reassure the client that there is no "pass or fail." There are many different ways to practice relaxation, and it's important to identify the techniques most beneficial for the client and modify the practice so that it's most helpful given the individual client's specific symptom presentation and needs.

- **"I don't have time. I'm just too busy to relax."** Explain that reserving time to relax will enhance the client's long-term productivity and quality of life. These skills help us better manage the stressors of a demanding life and schedule. With relaxation, we can reduce the amount of time we spend in acute distress and minimize the impact of stress on daily functioning and well-being. The time the client devotes to relaxation practice will decrease over time, as they become more familiar with the strategies. While it's best to start out by setting aside a time to practice in a quiet place, over time the client will be able to practice "on the go" without taking additional time out of their schedule.

- **"The problem is that I'm relaxing all the time; that's all I do!"** This may especially be the case for clients with post-COVID-19 fatigue or mobility limitations. Explain that although relaxation may feel like a passive activity, it is an active behavioral approach with an established physiological target and benefit. It has benefit even for those with chronic fatigue and chronic pain with diminished activity tolerance. Relaxation is very different from resting, lounging, or enjoying a hobby. Relaxation requires work, persistence, and behaving with intention. Unlike when we're resting or lounging, relaxation strategies produce physiological changes that help to reduce hyperarousal and tension, and they improve our ability to manage stress.

■ **"I want to learn the skills, but I'm having trouble remembering to practice."** This is a common problem and can be even more pronounced among clients experiencing residual cognitive difficulties post-COVID-19. Normalize this for the client. Explain that creating a new habit can be very difficult and is hardest to implement in the beginning. Then, problem-solve strategies to increase engagement, modified to the specific needs of the client. Along with collaboratively making a plan with the client using Worksheet 6.5: My Relaxation Plan, use digital and visual reminders and enlist support from family members and loved ones.

Worksheet 6.1
Self-Soothing Skills

Self-soothing and distraction can help to shift your focus away from the stressor and increase feelings of relaxation. The purpose of this worksheet is to identify effective self-soothing and distraction techniques that might be particularly helpful for you to alleviate acute stress and reduce the emotional intensity of the moment.

> **Remember**: Without practice, these strategies are difficult to apply when they're needed most (e.g., when you're feeling a strong emotion or high level of stress). Begin by practicing your selected skills for a few minutes every day during non-stressful moments, for at least a few weeks. Regular practice will make these skills more effective and easier to use in times of need.

Self-Soothing Using the Five Senses

Using the five senses can help to pull your attention away from the stressor and refocus on aspects of the physical world. This anchors your attention to the present moment. Below is a list of self-soothing strategies involving the five senses. Evoking different sensations creates space from your internal thoughts and directs your attention to something other than the emotional distress and its source.

- **Sight**: Focus your attention and energy on what's visible in the present moment. What do you see? What catches your eye? Notice its various details and features (colors, contours, shades). It can help to identify several soothing things to observe like a painting, or pictures of nature, loved ones, pets, a favorite vacation spot, or place of comfort. Change the environment, go outdoors, or go to a soothing indoor space.
- **Touch**: Select an item. It can be either a soothing grounding item or anything within your reach (like a pen). Gently run your fingers over it, and take a moment to direct your full attention to its features and components. What do you notice? Take note of the texture, smoothness, contours, heaviness, lightness, softness, and so on. Introducing different temperatures can quickly lessen your stress response and shift your attention to the present moment. For instance, take a warm shower or bath, or rub an ice cube on your hands, face, chest, or forearms.
- **Smell**: Smells can have a powerful effect on your mood. Identify smells that put you at ease or give you a sense of comfort, or that you find pleasant (lavender, vanilla, cinnamon, baked cookies). Other examples are scented candles, body or hand lotions, and certain foods or spices.

- **Sound**: Identify sounds that have a calming effect or bring on positive feelings, and focus your attention on what you hear. Examples include sound machines or mobile apps with nature sounds (ocean, rain), loud or upbeat music, songs that remind you of a pleasant memory, or listening to a taped prayer or mantra.
- **Taste**: Select items to engage your sense of taste, such as a soothing drink (herbal tea, hot chocolate), peppermint gum, or a piece of chocolate. Do so mindfully, directing your full attention to really focus on the taste of the item.

Examples of Self-Soothing Using the Five Senses

SEE	HEAR
☐ Notice the nature around you, even outside the window; search for things you haven't noticed before	☐ Listen to your specific sounds of comfort (nature sounds, music, audio of loved one's voice)
☐ Observe the clouds in the sky pass by	☐ Listen to soothing music
☐ Notice leaves on a tree move in the wind	☐ Open your window and listen to the sounds outside
☐ Walk in a park; take a scenic hike	☐ Play a mobile app, sound machine, or video of nature sounds (ocean waves, rainfall)
☐ Count colors in a painting	
☐ Watch the flame of a candle	☐ Listen to the radio or a podcast
☐ Look at a picture of a loved one, pet, or favorite place to visit/vacation spot	☐ Turn on a white noise machine
	☐ Listen to wind chimes
☐ Stream a video of nature (waterfall, ocean, rain forest)	☐ Play a recording of a prayer
☐ Change your environment from the source of distress (go outdoors or to a soothing indoor space)	☐ Listen to music that invigorates you, puts you in a positive mood, or reminds you of a fond memory
☐ Visit a nearby place you enjoy (museum, park)	
Other_____	Other_____
Other_____	Other_____

TOUCH

- ☐ Take a hot or cold shower
- ☐ Touch a comforting home item (soft blanket or sweater) or an item with special meaning
- ☐ Put cold compress/ice cubes on forehead, cheek, chest, hands, arms
- ☐ Pet a cat or dog
- ☐ Hug or hold hands with a loved one
- ☐ Squeeze a rubber/stress ball
- ☐ Touch a grounding item (seashell, smooth rock) and notice its features (textures, weight, temperature)
- ☐ Do gentle stretching

Other_____

Other _____

TASTE

- ☐ Put an ice cube in your mouth
- ☐ Drink a glass of cold water
- ☐ Drink herbal tea or hot chocolate
- ☐ Savor a piece of chocolate
- ☐ Chew gum or a mint
- ☐ Enjoy a favorite food

Other_____

Other _____

SMELL

- ☐ Use scented body/hand lotion
- ☐ Light a scented candle
- ☐ Smell coffee grounds
- ☐ Make popcorn or cookies
- ☐ Smell fresh flowers
- ☐ Open the window; breathe in crisp, fresh air outside
- ☐ Use essential oils (lavender, chamomile, citrus)
- ☐ Use an oil diffuser
- ☐ Smell vanilla, cinnamon, or other spices

Other_____

Other _____

Worksheet 6.2
Soothing Self-Statements

Choose one or a few short, self-soothing statements that resonate with you. In moments of acute stress, you can repeat these over and over, out loud or silently. Self-soothing statements can be done alone or paired with another relaxation strategy, like deep breathing.

"This feeling is temporary, this moment is temporary, I can get through this."
"I'm safe and secure in this moment."
"I'm going to focus on what I can do, not what I can't."
"I've gotten through difficult times before and I can get through this one too."
"There are skills I can use to cope."
"This emotion won't last forever."
"I control where my attention is, and I can focus on something else."
"I'm doing my best, and I can ride this out."
"I'm strong, and I can move through this painful moment."

Along with the examples above, identify other reminders or self-statements that might be particularly helpful to you during difficult moments. Also make note of any inspirational quotes, mantras, or prayers that are particularly meaningful to you.

*Other*_____

Other _____

Other _____

Physical exercise:

☐ Stretch

☐ Go for a walk outside

☐ Yoga

☐ Gardening or yardwork

☐ Walk your dog/play with your pet

☐ Swim

Cognitive exercise:

☐ Read a book

☐ Puzzles

☐ Sudoku

☐ Crosswords

☐ Computer games

☐ Play cards or other games (mah-jongg, bridge, etc.)

Shift your attention to an easy task on your to-do list:

☐ Laundry

☐ Dishes

☐ Vacuuming

☐ Clean a room/corner in your house

☐ Repair or fix something

☐ Start or finish a project

☐ Decorate or rearrange your house

Give back:

☐ Volunteer

☐ Surprise someone with something nice

☐ Help a loved one or neighbor

☐ Do something thoughtful for someone else (make a meal for a neighbor)

☐ Reach out to a loved one going through hardship, send an encouraging message, or just say hello

☐ Collect clothes/items to donate

Activities that provide a sense of joy or comfort:

☐ Cook

☐ Call or video chat with a friend or loved one

☐ Go outside and sit in the sun

☐ Play an instrument

☐ Engage in hobbies (gardening, painting, woodworking)

☐ Pray, repeat a mantra

☐ Watch a comedy, movie, or show you know creates pleasant feelings

Worksheet 6.4
Relaxation Practice Record

Date	Relaxation Skill Used	Stress Before Practice (1–10)	Stress After Practice (1–10)

Worksheet 6.5
My Relaxation Plan

It is helpful to have a **selection of relaxation strategies** that you can use at various times and in various circumstances. Identify the strategies you've found to be most effective for you. Create a plan for which ones you want to use in which setting. Relaxation exercises may include breathing-based relaxation (diaphragmatic breathing); imagery; and self-soothing strategies, including using the five senses, calming self-statements, and distracting activities.

At home:

1. _____

2. _____

3. _____

4. _____

5. _____

Out or "on the go":

1. _____

2. _____

3. _____

4. _____

5. _____

In a rush, or only have a few minutes:

1. _____

2. _____

3. _____

4. _____

5. _____

CHAPTER 7

Module 7: Reframing Unhelpful Thoughts

Chapter Overview

In this chapter, clients will learn skills for observing unhelpful thoughts, reframing unhelpful thoughts, and responding to thoughts more effectively. Clients will be introduced to the concept of helpful and unhelpful thoughts, learn strategies to modify unhelpful thoughts, and practice self-validating non-distorted thoughts. The worksheets include a list of common thinking traps and an automatic thought record.

Number of Sessions

We recommend spending at least three sessions on this chapter. Consider administering self-report symptom questionnaires (e.g., PHQ-9, GAD-7) at the beginning of the session to continue tracking symptoms of depression and anxiety.

Therapeutic Content

Introduction

For clients who have developed depressive or anxious symptoms after contracting COVID-19, it is common for certain physical symptoms such as fatigue, shortness of breath, cognitive symptoms, or mobility problems to trigger unhelpful thoughts, such as "I'm never going to get better" or "I'll never be able to function the way I did before." These thoughts might also be triggered by observing others engage in behaviors the client used to be able to do with ease, having to ask others for help while engaging in day-to-day activities, or having to stop and rest in response to fatigue while out in public. Clients may respond to these thoughts with maladaptive behaviors, such as avoiding physical therapy appointments or avoiding asking for help.

By *unhelpful thoughts*, we refer to thoughts, interpretations, and beliefs that may be accurate to varying degrees but perpetuate negative emotions and avoidance behaviors that keep the client stuck and prevent them from fully engaging in recovery and rehabilitation to lead a fulfilling life despite ongoing COVID-19 symptoms. While the physical sensations or environmental triggers for the client's unhelpful thoughts may be outside of their scope of control, we teach them that by modifying unhelpful thoughts, they can lessen the intensity of painful emotions, better engage in day-to-day activities, and improve their overall functioning. The practice of reframing unhelpful thought patterns, as practiced in cognitive therapy and cognitive behavioral therapy (CBT), has been shown to effectively reduce symptoms of depression and anxiety, as well as other mental health challenges (Chambless & Gillis, 1993; Scott, 2001).

Thinking Traps

Some individuals may develop and become attached to unhelpful interpretations in response to events. For example, if an employee, Sara, is called to a meeting by her boss, she might interpret this to mean that she has done something wrong and will soon be fired. This pattern of thought is referred to as a "thinking trap" or "cognitive distortion" in traditional CBT treatment. Thinking traps occur when an individual gets stuck on one automatic interpretation of an otherwise ambiguous event, which can often reflect a "worst-case scenario" outcome. Thinking traps can exacerbate painful emotions like sadness or anxiety. The intensity of Sara's resultant anxiety could be significantly reduced if she were able to practice "cognitive flexibility" and explore alternative interpretations of this event. For example, Sara could interpret her boss's request for a meeting as a potential opportunity for the boss to share their own personal news with her, or possibly discuss a promotion for Sara, or provide neutral or even positive feedback to Sara on her recent work.

Clients who are experiencing persistent sequelae of COVID-19 will likely also have thoughts surrounding their uncertain prognosis and the possibility that their physical symptoms will persist. To reduce distress related to uncertainty, you will encourage clients to come up with helpful thoughts that acknowledge uncertainty without added distortion. For example, teaching clients to reframe "fortune telling" thoughts like "This is never going to get better" into valid thoughts that reflect uncertainty, such as "I'm not sure when I will physically feel the way I did before contracting COVID-19, but if I keep working at it I have a better chance," can lessen the intensity of painful emotions and feelings of hopelessness and motivate actions toward the client's goals.

Therapist Note

Many clients, as well as therapists newer to CBT, interpret the concept of reframing unhelpful thoughts to mean that the goal is "positive thinking." Inform clients that the goal of reframing unhelpful thoughts is not simply to think positively but rather to aim for balanced, flexible, and helpful thinking that motivates the client to work toward their goals, recovery, and rehabilitation.

Psychoeducation on Unhelpful Thoughts and Their Association with Emotions and Behaviors

At this point in treatment, you will already be familiar with your client's presenting challenges, including the persisting sequelae of COVID-19 they continue to struggle with and their associated emotions. Use this information to begin the discussion of identifying triggers to unhelpful thoughts, identifying the content of their unhelpful thoughts, and teaching the skills to reframe those thoughts.

Begin this chapter by reviewing psychoeducational materials surrounding the CBT model of psychotherapy. Using Worksheet 2.1: Cognitive Behavioral Model, provided in Chapter 2, review the relationship between the client's physical/medical symptoms, distressing emotions, unhelpful thoughts, unhelpful behaviors, and the interplay between these factors. Case Vignette 7.1 is an example of how to provide psychoeducation.

THERAPIST: *To better understand the relationship between situations, thoughts, and behaviors, and our overall emotional functioning, imagine a person, Sam, in this situation. Sam sees his friend Marco on the street and waves hello, but Marco keeps walking and does not wave back. Sam then thinks, "Marco must not like me. I bet none of my friends really like me or want to spend time with me." Can you imagine how Sam might feel if he had that thought?*

CLIENT: *Probably really sad, or maybe a little anxious about his other relationships.*

THERAPIST: *Exactly. That type of thought reflects a bit of mind reading, as though Sam has the power to read other people's thoughts. It also reflects generalization, as though Sam's experiences with one person are the same as his experiences with other people. In a little while we're going to talk more about mind reading, and generalization, as well as other traps people often fall into with their thinking patterns.*

CLIENT: *OK, and I definitely have fallen into the mind-reading habit, and assumed that people were mad at me, even if they never said that.*

THERAPIST: *Exactly; many people have! And let's say if Sam has this thought, how helpful is it for him to have that thought if we imagine he is a person who values his friendships and social connections?*

CLIENT: *It's probably not too helpful. He's making an assumption. It would probably lead to him not wanting to speak with Marco anymore. He might stay away from other friends too.*

THERAPIST: *That's right. Now let's say that Sam does in fact isolate himself from Marco and his other friends. Can you imagine what's likely to happen to that feeling of sadness?*

CLIENT: *It'll probably feel a lot worse.*

THERAPIST: *Yes, that's likely. That feeling of sadness would likely persist into a worse, longstanding low mood. However, if Sam had a different thought in response to that event, or if he were able to reframe that thought to a more helpful one, like "Maybe Marco was in a rush," Sam would likely feel differently.*

CLIENT: *Yeah, that makes sense. He probably would be less likely to isolate or feel sad or anxious.*

THERAPIST: *Exactly! The interpretation "Maybe Marco was in a rush" is a more helpful thought because it helped move Sam closer to the life he wants to lead. OK, now let's use an example closer to some of your challenges. A person might struggle with shortness of breath after contracting COVID-19, even several weeks or months after their initial infection, and have the thought "This is never going to get better." Can you imagine how that person is likely to feel in response to that thought?*

CLIENT: *I've definitely had that thought. It's made me feel terrible, really sad, scared, and kind of hopeless.*

THERAPIST: *I can completely understand that and also understand how hard that's been on you. How helpful is that thought for you? When that thought comes up for you, what do you find yourself doing?*

CLIENT: *Well, I've definitely skipped appointments before when I've felt that way, since I started thinking "What's the point anyway?" And I might spend the whole day in bed when I get really down. It's not very helpful for me to think like that, to be honest.*

THERAPIST: *And how have you felt after doing so?*

CLIENT: *Even worse, honestly.*

THERAPIST: *So if there was a way to reframe the thought that "This is never going to get better" to a more helpful thought, like "I'm not sure when my breathing will start coming easier. However, I can still follow my doctor's recommendations to try to improve these symptoms, and also do what I am still able to do," can you imagine how you might feel then?*

CLIENT: *Maybe still anxious, but maybe not as depressed.*

THERAPIST: *Exactly. You may not feel entirely better after reframing some of your unhelpful thoughts, but this can help you engage in more helpful behaviors and lessen how intense your painful emotions feel and shorten how long they last for.*

CLIENT: *Got it. So basically, I'll be practicing thinking positively? Because that usually doesn't work for me.*

THERAPIST: *Not exactly, and I'm not surprised it doesn't! People so commonly recommend that others simply "think positively" to feel better. Yet very rarely does forcing yourself to have more positive thoughts help, because these "positive thoughts" can feel false and even untrue! Telling yourself that you will probably feel back to 100 percent tomorrow is likely not going to make you feel better or be helpful to you, because it is unrealistic. Instead, we are going to practice generating more balanced beliefs, rather than thinking in extremes. An example of this would be learning to say to yourself, "I may not feel better tomorrow, and I don't know if or when I'll feel the way I did before catching COVID-19. But I have improved somewhat from the point of my initial infection, and there's a chance I'll continue to improve if I follow my medical team's recommendations."*

Next, use an example from the client's life to further explore unhelpful thoughts and their associations with COVID-19 symptoms, emotions, and behaviors. Examples of unhelpful thoughts that can emerge in the context of COVID-19 include "I will never get any better than this,"

"I'll never be able to live a normal life," or "I can't live a normal life until these feelings go away." After discussing your client's thoughts, work together to identify the behaviors they engage in. For example, clients might cancel or avoid medical appointments due to concern that their functioning will never improve, or clients might avoid leaving their home due to concern that they may lose their breath or develop fatigue and need to stop and rest. Collaborate with the client to identify the behaviors they engage in that likely negatively impact their emotional functioning.

Identifying Thinking Traps

Introduce the concept of "thinking traps" to the client. Explain that sometimes thoughts are unhelpful because our brain thinks in certain patterns that lead us to not see the fuller picture or keep us feeling stuck. Importantly, we all sometimes fall into thinking traps, as suggested by the relatively benign example above of a friend not responding. In the context of an illness like COVID-19, we may be more prone to falling into certain thinking traps around our beliefs for recovery and rehabilitation. With the client, read through Worksheet 7.1: Common Thinking Traps. Worksheets can be found at the end of this chapter in both the Therapist Guide and Client Workbook or can be accessed by searching for this book's title on the Oxford Academic platform, at academic.oup.com.

Identify any cognitive patterns that appear familiar and contribute to the client's distress. As you go through the list, ask the client to circle or check off ones they have noticed apply to them. This might include observations of "fortune telling" or predicting that in the future one's circumstances will never improve. Another example might include "discounting the positives" and dismissing areas of progress that the client has made because they still compare themselves to how they were before contracting COVID-19.

Highlight to the client that many thoughts contain a grain of truth, and we are not saying that the thought is necessarily inaccurate. For example, one might have the thought "Everyone in my life fails to respond to me when I feel alone." In actuality, some of this person's loved ones might decline their calls or cancel plans, but the way this is described as "everyone" may reflect a pattern of unhelpful generalizing and all-or-nothing thinking and lead to increased feelings of sadness or resentment. Rather than accuracy, we are focusing on the helpfulness of the thought toward the client's goals.

Also clarify for the client that not every thought has to contain a thinking trap. For example, the thought "Many tasks are harder for me than they used to be" is a balanced, accurate, and nonjudgmental observation of their functioning. Other thoughts may reflect ongoing uncertainty, such as "I have no idea when I'm going to start feeling the way that I used to" or "I don't know if I will get COVID-19 again, and if I do, how that will affect my symptoms." These are examples of thoughts that likely do not contain thinking traps and do not necessarily need to be reframed. Rather, the thought can be validated as an expression of the client's ongoing struggles and uncertainty. In such situations, it can be fruitful to have the client mindfully acknowledge the thought and add a helpful, motivating statement at the end of the thought. For example, the client might say "I have no idea when I'm going to start feeling the way that I used to, and there are things I can do now to give myself a sense of enjoyment and maximize my odds of recovery." Or "I don't know if I will get COVID-19 again, but I can use certain measures to decrease my risk while making sure I'm safely participating in the activities that matter most to me." To distinguish between balanced thoughts and thoughts with thinking traps, look for extremes in the client's language. These include words like "always," "never," and "should."

Reframing Unhelpful Thoughts

Once the client has described their thoughts, introduce them to Worksheet 7.2: Automatic Thought Record and the use of guided questions to reframe thoughts. Go through an example in session using the following steps to reframe unhelpful thoughts:

1. Thinks of a situation or trigger.
2. Notice any automatic, unhelpful thoughts that come up.
3. Rate their emotion.
4. Note any thinking traps that they might have fallen into.

5. Use guided questions to probe for alternate explanations or possibilities.
6. Come up with a balanced, helpful thought in response to the initial automatic thought.
7. Rate emotions again.

Use Socratic, guided questioning to help the client come up with alternate possibilities and balanced, helpful thoughts. Example statements can include: *"What is the evidence this thought is true? What is the evidence this thought is not true? Is there another possible explanation or perspective? How helpful is it for you to have that automatic thought? Does that automatic thought move you closer to or farther away from your goals for recovery? Does that automatic thought move you closer to or farther away from engaging in the activities that are meaningful to you? What's an alternate and more helpful thought you can have?"*

Therapist Note

It may be unrealistic to expect that the client will have significant change in their emotions after reframing their thoughts, at least early on. Highlight to the client that even if there is no or minimal change in emotional intensity, coming up with helpful thoughts can still motivate more adaptive behaviors. Explain that with practice, emotional intensity may decrease.

At-Home Practice

After completing an entry on Worksheet 7.2: Automatic Thought Record in session, guide the client to plan when and in what situations they would practice responding to an unhelpful thought with their reframed helpful thought. Ask the client, "If the situation occurs again, what would you want to tell yourself?" to encourage rehearsal of these more helpful thoughts in future similar events (Beck, 2020). You can also instruct the client to repeat aloud or to themselves their reframing statement as a practice of more helpful self-talk. Explain that the more the client practices responding to unhelpful thoughts with helpful thoughts, the easier it will become to do so over the long term. Instruct the client to daily read their reframes from their Thought Records. Anchor this to a particular time (i.e., reading through their Thought Records in the mornings, or in the evenings) and instruct clients to read their reframes as needed throughout the day.

Self-Validation of Thoughts Related to Uncertainty

As discussed above, some thoughts that lead to the client's emotional distress might not involve the presence of any thinking traps, but rather reflect valid uncertainty surrounding their COVID-19 symptoms, functioning, and prognosis. For example, many clients present to this program with worries surrounding when their physical symptoms will remit to the point that they can return to previous employment positions or recreational activities (or if they ever will). In this case, we recommend that you validate the discomfort that comes along with sitting with such uncertainty. Clients may also benefit from practicing self-validating statements, which were introduced in Chapter 3. In response to a painful and recurrent automatic thought that your client might be having, encourage the client to observe the thought and label it. The client might say to themselves, for example, "I'm having the thought that I'm not going to be able to return to my job." You can encourage your client to try closing their eyes and saying to themselves, "It makes sense that I'm having this thought" or "Most other people would also have this thought in this situation." Even without reframing thoughts, labeling and self-validating thoughts can help the client move to choosing actions and behaviors that are closer to their goals, despite the presence of unhelpful thoughts. It can also create distance from the thought so that the client does not feel as stuck in it.

Practicing self-validation for thoughts related to the disproportionate impact of COVID-19 on marginalized groups is particularly important for ethnic and racial minority clients. Black and Hispanic American clients might present to treatment with feelings of sadness and anger connected to the unfairness involved with the disproportionate number of minority clients who have died from COVID-19, as well as limited vaccines that were made available to minorities during the initial vaccine rollouts. We strongly encourage validating those thoughts, and encouraging clients to validate their own distress, rather than attempting to reframe these thoughts or evaluate them any differently.

Pairing self-validation with relaxation skills taught in Chapter 6 may help lower the intensity of emotions that coincide with these valid concerns. For example, while using a self-validating statement such as described above, the client can be guided to simultaneously practice diaphragmatic breathing to lessen the intensity of their anxiety as needed. Finally, if a client's perception of their situation is valid and leads to distress, investigate whether there is an avenue for problem-solving to address their difficulties. For example, given uncertainty about a client's future functioning due to COVID-19, problem-solving might involve asking for help from family members as needed to lessen the potential financial burden of a change in employment.

Worksheet 7.1
Common Thinking Traps*

We all fall into these thinking traps from time to time—it's the way our brains naturally process information. However, thought patterns like these often lead us to feel stuck, contribute to difficult emotions, and make it less likely that we will act in a way that moves us toward our goals.

Read through this worksheet and identify any of the thinking patterns that you have been falling into lately.

1. **Mind Reading**: You assume that you know what people think without having sufficient evidence of their thoughts. Examples: "That person is annoyed with me because I am walking slowly in front of them," "Other people don't believe that I feel as sick as I do."
2. **Fortune Telling**: You predict the future—that things will get worse or that there is danger ahead. Examples: "I'm never going to be able to go back to work," "I'll never feel better."
3. **Catastrophizing or Thinking the Worst**: You believe that what has happened or will happen will be so awful and unbearable that you won't be able to stand it: "I'm going to get COVID-19 again and have to go back to the hospital."
4. **Discounting the Positives**: You claim that the positive accomplishments you attain are trivial: "Even though I've made a little progress in my COVID-19 symptoms, it doesn't matter because I still feel terrible."
5. **Overgeneralizing**: You perceive a global pattern of negatives based on a single incident: "The last treatment my doctor recommended didn't work, so I know this one won't work, either."
6. **Black-and-White Thinking**: You view events, or people, in all-or-nothing terms. Examples: "If I don't get back to exactly the way I was, I will never be happy," "If I don't start feeling back to normal, my life is worthless."
7. **"Should" Statements**: You interpret events in terms of how things should be rather than simply focusing on what is: "I should be feeling better by now! Everyone else I know who's gotten COVID does."

Adapted from Leahy, R. L. (1996). *Cognitive therapy: Basic principles and applications.* Northvale.

Worksheet 7.2
Automatic Thought Record

Questions to help you generate alternate, helpful thoughts: What evidence do you have for the thought? What evidence do you have against the thought? Is there another possible explanation, perspective, or outcome? How helpful is it for you to have this thought? Does that automatic thought move you closer to or farther away from attaining your goals for recovery and engaging in activities that are meaningful to you?

Situation (Trigger)	Automatic Thought	Emotion	Thinking Trap(s)	Alternate, Helpful Thought	Re-rate Emotion

CHAPTER 8

Module 8: Confronting Feared and Avoided Situations

Chapter Overview

The purpose of this chapter is to evaluate with clients the function of avoidance in their lives, to identify any existing maladaptive avoidance behaviors and patterns, and to encourage and practice engaging in avoided situations to reduce anxiety and to improve functioning. Two worksheets are provided in this chapter—Worksheet 8.1: Identifying Avoidance and Its Consequences and Worksheet 8.2: Engaging in Avoided Activities.

Number of Sessions

You will want to spend anywhere between one and three sessions on this chapter with clients, depending on the clinical presentation of the client and the extent of avoidance behaviors. Consider administering self-report symptom questionnaires (e.g., PHQ-9, GAD-7) at the beginning of the session to continue tracking symptoms of depression and anxiety.

> **Therapist Note**
> *This chapter is not intended to be an exhaustive protocol for exposure therapy; clients who meet diagnostic criteria for panic disorder, specific phobia, obsessive-compulsive disorder, or other psychiatric disorder in which exposure-based treatment is warranted may benefit from dedicated exposure protocols for these conditions (Kaczkurkin & Foa, 2022).*

Psychoeducation

The Consequences of Avoidance

Review with the client that in response to something frightening, we experience an urge or instinct to avoid or escape that feared stimulus. This urge is due to our fight-or-flight reaction, first discussed in Chapter 3 and further elaborated on in Chapter 6. While this response is innate and adaptive when we are in dangerous situations, sometimes the fight-or-flight system is activated in situations that are not inherently dangerous, or that are no longer dangerous. The key point for this chapter is that the fight-or-flight system motivates avoidance and escape. In this chapter, we will explore how clients who contracted COVID-19 may develop fears of both internal and external stimuli that lead to unhelpful avoidance and escape behaviors. We will also explain the value of reducing those avoidance behaviors through engaging with feared and avoided situations in a safe, graded manner.

Here are some ways in which fear and avoidance may be experienced by individuals recovering from COVID-19:

- After attending a group gathering where the client contracted COVID-19, they come to fear and avoid social gatherings.
- They continue to avoid leaving their home for fear of encountering others, which is how they contracted COVID-19. Even "safer activities" (interacting with vaccinated others while vaccinated, engaging in outdoor distanced activities) are avoided, leading to social isolation and worsening mood.
- The avoidance generalizes to medical appointments and other necessary visits and becomes maladaptive for the client who is now not engaging in medical care.
- The client may start to engage in excessive reassurance seeking—which can be conceptualized as a form of avoidance—that can lead to excessive monitoring of physical signs beyond what has been recommended medically.

Triggers, illustrated above using social situations as a paradigm, can extend to any stimuli that have become associated with illness. For instance, the experience of shortness of breath, which is a familiar phenomenon for anyone who has gone up a flight of stairs, can become a trigger for the fight-or-flight response after COVID-19. Similarly, even after the acute period of the client's COVID-19 symptoms has passed, they might develop patterns of avoiding triggers even remotely associated with shortness of breath that now may give rise to uncomfortable emotions. Such triggers can include physical movement and fluctuations in pain and fatigue.

Differentiating False Alarms from True Alarms

It is important for you to have a thorough understanding of your client's current, objective medical status. This understanding can draw from your client's self-report and your case conceptualization, from available medical records, and from discussion with the client's primary care physician or other medical providers. This knowledge will help you differentiate "true alarms" from "false alarms," and adaptive avoidance behaviors from maladaptive avoidance behaviors. By true alarms versus false alarms, we refer to situations in which anxiety or fear may be valid, as compared to times in which the anxiety and fear is out of proportion to the threat or does not actually signify a threat.

For example, a client with residual physical/medical symptoms of COVID-19 who is asked to monitor their oxygen using a pulse oximeter likely has specific instructions from their physician as to the fluctuations that are normal compared to those that are abnormal and warrant concern. If Client A has been told that fluctuations to a certain threshold (as an example, "90") are not cause for concern, then anxiety-driven avoidance upon seeing a reading of "96" can be conceptualized as a "false alarm." On the other hand, if Client B has been told that a reading of "90" is abnormal and signifies they should rest or seek medical attention sees a reading of "90" and experiences anxiety, that is a valid and true alarm that warrants a different course of action such as resting or notifying their provider or other emergency response.

Clients recovering from COVID-19 may have guidelines from their providers regarding recommended levels of activity and exertion. Note that the medical status and functional capabilities of a client often evolve over time from the initial infection. As illustrated in Case Vignette 8.1, what may have been an adaptive avoidance behavior can morph into a maladaptive behavior over time. It can even revert into an adaptive behavior if further medical complications arise. Communication with providers and access to medical records can help you determine to what extent your client may be engaging in maladaptive avoidance.

Case Vignette 8.1

Arlene is a 39-year-old female, presenting for treatment of anxiety that developed following a debilitating battle with COVID-19. She was discharged from the hospital with instructions to remain home until her symptoms remitted, and to monitor her symptoms with a pulse oximeter. However, even after Arlene's acute symptoms abated, she continued to observe some tightness in her chest with activities of mild to moderate intensity, as well as intermittent and unpredictable bouts of tachycardia. Her doctors prescribed monitoring of her oxygen levels every 8 hours until her symptoms improved. Gradually her chest tightness improved, and her oxygen levels consistently read in the normal range. Her doctor cleared her to resume daily activities and told her it was no longer necessary to monitor her oxygen. However, Arlene continued to track her oxygen levels on an hourly basis and call her doctor frantically whenever her levels transiently dipped below "97" long after her symptoms improved. She also continued to largely avoid leaving her home. She would experience immense difficulty attending her medical visits and insisted on virtual visits, and even refused to attend physical therapy appointments. Her mood worsened as she grew to miss socializing with her loved ones. She transitioned jobs to one that was entirely remote in order to avoid face-to-face contact. She describes to her therapist that she feels as though she has "an entirely different life now," and that she misses her old one but is too afraid to try to get it back.

Excessive Checking and Self-Monitoring as a Form of Avoidance

We have found in our work with clients with persistent symptoms of COVID-19 that avoidance does not always take the form of withdrawal from an activity or sensation, but can sometimes manifest as excessive checking of, and hypervigilance to, medical and physical symptoms. This can be conceptualized as another form of avoidance, where the fear of having a physical setback or medical decline is the emotion that is being avoided. This form of avoidance may be present in those individuals with a more complicated and severe hospital course.

Targeting this form of avoidance works in an analogous manner as targeting avoidance that encompasses withdrawal from activities or sensations. You and the client should note what a reasonable amount of checking or vigilance to medical symptoms is—this can often be guided by medical recommendations, such as in Case Vignette 8.1, where the client was instructed to take a pulse oximeter reading at a certain frequency by her physician. Point out the short-term and long-term consequences of excessive checking and hypervigilance, which typically result in immediate but temporary feelings of reassurance and relief, but in the long term fuel and perpetuate the emotion of fear. The goal should then be to prevent checking and symptom monitoring that is more than recommended by a client's medical providers.

Identifying Avoidance and Its Consequences

Once your client has a grasp of the concepts of avoidance and exposure, proceed to Worksheet 8.1: Identifying Avoidance and Its Consequences in session. Worksheets can be found at the end of this chapter in both the Therapist Guide and Client Workbook or can be accessed by searching for this book's title on the Oxford Academic platform, at academic.oup.com.

Worksheet 8.1 helps clarify situations and physical sensations that the client is currently avoiding, whether that avoidance is adaptive or maladaptive (i.e., whether it is medically indicated), the distress that that situation would cause if the activity was engaged in, and the functional consequences of avoidance. At the top of the worksheet, it can be helpful to write any medically or physically based activity restrictions or limitations, as well as current public health guidance around COVID-19, to determine whether the client's level of avoidance is appropriate and adaptive, or maladaptive.

In session, ask the client to describe activities or physical sensations they may currently be avoiding. Ask the client how emotionally distressing they anticipate these activities to be. Avoidance may center around an upcoming rehabilitation session or medical procedure, social activity, physical exertion, or another situation. Avoidance can also center around physical sensations, such as avoidance of any activity that increases shortness of breath or heart rate, or that may cause fatigue. As in other exposure protocols, distress can be quantified using a Subjective Units of Distress Scale (or SUDS) in the second column. Ask the client to rate on a 0-to-10 scale how emotionally distressing they imagine the avoided activity to be. A zero rating represents the complete absence of emotional distress or discomfort. A 10 rating represents the most emotionally distressing or uncomfortable situation imaginable. These ratings can be useful to rank order situations that your client can engage in in a graded fashion.

In the third and fourth columns, ask your client to describe separately the short-term and long-term consequences of avoidance. Consequences can encompass emotions (i.e., how the client feels after avoiding), thoughts, and material consequences (i.e., in terms of what happened to the client and/or others in the client's life). Often, there is a temporary and short-term benefit to avoidance. This can include feelings of relief, a sense of safety, and thoughts such as "I'm safe" or "I prevented myself from getting worse [or prevented some horrible catastrophe from happening]." These short-term benefits can reinforce and perpetuate further avoidance. However, avoidance usually has negative long-term consequences. These can include a continued feeling of anxiety or fear, diminished social interaction and/or engagement in valued and meaningful activities, and worse long-term medical and physical prognosis (if the client has avoided medical care or rehabilitation). Helping your client to explore long-term consequences can underscore the maladaptive consequences of avoidance and can boost the client's motivation to practice engaging in avoided situations and confronting their fears.

In the fifth column, discuss and explore with your client whether avoidance (and the avoided activity or sensation) is reasonable based on the client's medical and physical restrictions and limitations, as well as with current public health guidelines related to the COVID-19 pandemic. In the sixth column, probe how important or meaningful the activity is to your client. This exercise helps decision-making regarding reasonable versus potentially harmful activities to engage in. At times, there may be clear "yes" or "no" answers to this question. For example, a client avoids driving under the guidance of her physician, who tells her she is not yet recovered enough to safely drive; or a client who has been told by his physician that he can resume all activities as normal may nevertheless refrain from exercising or exerting himself. At other times, there will not be a clear "yes" or "no" answer. This can be especially true in the case of fear of reinfection and avoidance of situations in which the client may be at elevated risk of re-contracting COVID-19. If the answer to the question is that the client is unsure, then it is particularly important to explore the information in Column 6—that is, how important, valued, and meaningful that activity is to the client, and how much not engaging in it interferes with their life. If the client identifies the activity as important and valued, then you can work with them to problem-solve ways in which they can engage in the activity while balancing the mitigation of COVID-19 infection risk.

Preparing the Client to Confront Feared and Avoided Situations

Now that you and the client have identified situations that the client is avoiding that are safe for them to engage in (medically and physically), provide psychoeducation on the rationale for confronting feared and avoided situations:

"When you repeatedly confront and engage in avoided situations where fear is a false alarm, a couple of helpful psychological processes happen. The first can be 'habituation,' where you may notice that the fear and intensity decrease over time the more you engage in the activity or situation. Your brain starts to learn that the situation is not (or is no longer) threatening. Your fight-or-flight system response may go down, which we see in Figure 8.1. This is an example of a client who experienced fear and distress anytime he planned to do home physical therapy. He avoided his exercises because he feared a negative consequence. He also feared that the intensity of his emotions would be unbearable and that his fear would make him "go crazy." The first time he attempted to do a home physical therapy exercise, his fear level was quite high. But he stuck with the exercise and noted that he felt less afraid (and even a bit proud!) at the end of it. The next day he tried the home physical therapy exercise, and he noticed that his fear was not quite as high. Again, his fear diminished as he practiced his exercises."

This reduction in emotional distress and discomfort (usually fear) is what is called habituation. Habituation to a feared stimulus can occur when an individual repeatedly approaches non-threatening but

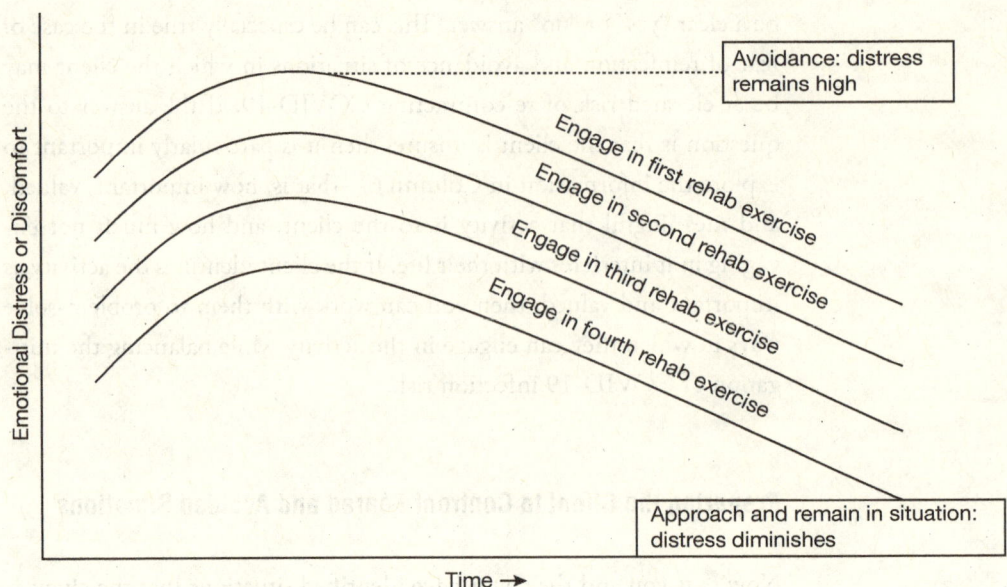

Figure 8.1.

Example of Habituation by Repeatedly Confronting an Avoided Situation

anxiety-provoking situations and their fear response decreases over time (Cornwell et al., 2013). However, habituation does not always happen. Sometimes, the emotional discomfort stays high, but new emotions are also felt, such as pride and accomplishment. Even if the emotional intensity does not go down, the client is still learning that that situation is tolerable and that their level of emotional intensity can be coped with. As shown in Case Vignette 8.2, clients can learn that periodic changes in their bodily sensations are not inherently dangerous when monitored as directed by their medical team.

Case Vignette 8.2

THERAPIST: *Hi, Arlene! As we get started with this portion of treatment, I want to start by asking: Have you ever been afraid of something that you aren't afraid of anymore?*

CLIENT: *Of course I have! I remember I used to be afraid of the dark when I was a kid. I also used to be terrified of driving.*

THERAPIST: *Really? Fear of the dark is so common in children. And I recall you saying you drive now, or at least that you used to, every day for work. So you're no longer afraid of driving?*

CLIENT: *Nope—I mean, I'm afraid of a lot of things these days, but driving isn't really one of them.*

THERAPIST: *Gotcha, and we'll come back to addressing some of those other things in a minute. But let me ask you first: How do you think you stopped becoming afraid of driving?*

CLIENT: *I don't really know. At some point my parents got sick of driving me around everywhere, and insisted I start driving for myself. I guess they kind of forced me into it, first by practicing with my dad in parking lots, then on quiet local roads, until I felt prepared to get my license. Then I just kept driving. When I got a job that was like 45 minutes away from home, I really started driving a lot. I guess it was around then that I stopped being afraid of it.*

THERAPIST: *That's interesting and is exactly what we're going to spend some time talking about today. It doesn't surprise me at all that your fear of driving didn't disappear into thin air one day. What you just described is a perfect example of how engaging in an activity that's scary leads to feeling less afraid over time. This is a therapeutic technique that has been well researched, called "exposure." It involves doing the things you are afraid of, rather than avoiding them, when the things you might be afraid of are not inherently dangerous and your doctor has said they're OK for you to do. When you do so, you might discover that the fear you experience with repeated practice goes down over time, kind of like your fear of driving decreased over time.*

CLIENT: *OK, I think I understand.*

THERAPIST: *Great! And in engaging in the things you're afraid of, even if that fear doesn't go down or it takes a long time to, you learn that you can still be in control over your behaviors and actions, and that your fear doesn't have to be in control of you.*

CLIENT: *I mean, that sounds great, and I do wish I had the power to do some of the things that I used to do. But I don't know if I'm ready to face my fears.*

THERAPIST: *I completely understand your hesitation. I will never force you to do anything you feel unwilling to try, nor will we ever have you practice confronting situations that are actually dangerous or that go against what your doctor or physical therapist has said is OK for you to do.*

CLIENT: *OK. That sounds better, I guess.*

Therapist Note

This portion of treatment can be difficult for clients to complete because it necessitates confronting feared situations. Clients must put themselves in situations in which anxiety, fear, distress, or discomfort might (temporarily) increase. For many clients, there will be a natural reluctance to avoid engaging in feared situations just as there are avoidance tendencies in the client's daily life. Exploring discrepancies between avoidance behaviors and the client's goals can help to enhance motivation to engage in exposure practice. Highlighting the long-term costs of avoidance, even with a short-term and temporary reduction in distress or discomfort, can be particularly important here. It can also be helpful to go back to the client's goals (Chapter 1) and the cognitive behavioral model (Chapter 2) to review and reinforce the long-term consequences of avoidance and to point out that avoidance does not bring the client closer to their goals. As we note above, make sure to differentiate between avoidance that is medically indicated and adaptive versus maladaptive avoidance, focusing on the latter.

Engaging in Avoided Activities

Once you and the client have a list of activities or sensations that are avoided, and the client agrees that the avoidance is unreasonable, out of proportion, or excessive, you can turn to setting an action plan for having the client practice engaging in that activity. Use Worksheet 8.2: Engaging in Avoided Activities. Worksheets can be found at the end of this chapter in both the Therapist Guide and Client Workbook or can be accessed by searching for this book's title on the Oxford Academic platform, at academic.oup.com.

It is usually best to start this exposure exercise with activities that the client anticipates will elicit a low to moderate level of distress. This makes the client more likely to remain in the situation and to gain self-efficacy and self-confidence. As a therapist, you also have a role to play in problem-solving strategies to help your client mitigate avoidance and stay in a situation. Come up with a plan for what the client can do if they experience an urge to avoid. First, review psychoeducation and remind them of their recovery goals. Recalling the reasons for why engaging in a particular avoided task is important and in line with the client's values and goals can help to motivate action and help the client think of the long-term costs of avoidance as opposed to focusing on the short-term relief from distress by avoiding. Relying on the psychoeducation you have provided, encourage the client to persist in completing the agreed-upon task.

If you have completed Chapter 7: Reframing Unhelpful Thoughts, then working with the client to create helpful, motivating thoughts when approaching the feared situation can be beneficial. For example, a client might create a balanced reappraisal and say to themselves: "This is going to be hard, but it's important for me to do it," "It makes sense that my anxiety is trying to alert me to a threat, but there is no danger right now," "I'm in a safe place to practice walking," or "I can handle this, and the anxiety won't go on forever." Clients sometimes find that visualizing themselves approaching the feared situation can facilitate the actual approach by improving self-confidence.

At-Home Practice

Assign the practice of engaging in that activity or situation for homework and ask the client to independently fill out the boxes on the worksheet after "Post-Activity." Encourage the client to use multiple worksheets if necessary. Review and reiterate the importance of at-home practice.

Physical Sensations and Interoceptive Anxiety

Many individuals recovering from COVID-19 experience interoceptive, somatic sensations (shortness of breath, dizziness, increased heart rate) and avoid activities that might bring these symptoms on. Relatedly, clients recovering from COVID-19 can also experience these physiological sensations in response to anxiety and distress. However, their distress is often magnified given the way many these symptoms mirror the real medical emergencies they might have faced after contracting COVID-19. Therefore, it is difficult for clients when facing these symptoms to not associate them with danger and an immediate (and occasionally maladaptive) behavior to escape those sensations. These escape behaviors might involve taking an anxiolytic medication, excessive use of pulse oximeters, calling their doctor for reassurance that their symptoms are not dangerous, or even visiting the emergency room. The client's life can easily become immersed in these avoidance behaviors.

In our work with clients with COVID-19, we have found that it is typically not necessary to deliberately induce those physical sensations. Oftentimes, physical sensations are present even when the client is at rest or engages in an activity of mild difficulty, although this can vary individually. Therefore, you can work with your client to identify those feared sensations and practice sitting with those sensations during session without escape, while rating any changes in SUDS levels as the exposure continues and the client does not avoid. We also recommend highlighting new learning that arises, even if SUDS levels do not decrease during a particular exposure practice. New learning might involve the client realizing that the symptoms dissipate in time, even without escape, and/or that the client is able to remain in control over their behaviors.

It is important to highlight here that some of the mindfulness practices described in Chapter 5 involve sitting with and observing physical sensations without escape, such as through practice of a body scan meditation. These practices can be brought into this chapter and practiced by allowing the client to observe, perhaps discomfort in their chest or elevated heart rates, while learning that this discomfort is not inherently dangerous and does not necessitate immediate and maladaptive escape.

Therapist Note

Many therapists will have previous experience implementing interoceptive exposures for clients presenting with panic disorder. This is because interoceptive exposure is a commonly practiced technique to help clients with panic disorder learn to tolerate and de-catastrophize physiological symptoms of anxiety and panic, and ultimately reduce avoidance of situations that might evoke those symptoms. These exposure practices often involve the direct induction of symptoms that are consistent with panic, such as mimicking shortness of breath by having clients breathe through a straw, or inducing dizziness by having the client spin around in a chair. Because the effect of interoceptive exposures in COVID-19 has not yet been researched and is not yet known, we do not recommend inducing symptoms of panic in this manner, unless the client's physical symptoms of COVID-19 have resolved, and you conceptualize your client as having panic disorder.

Special Considerations and Troubleshooting

As already mentioned in the introduction to this Therapist Guide, under the heading "Is This Treatment Program Right for You and Your Client?", make sure to assess whether the client meets criteria for PTSD in your initial intake assessment. PTSD presents with significant avoidance behaviors, and individuals with PTSD typically benefit from various forms of exposure practice, such as in vivo exposure to avoided situations that serve as reminders of past traumas, as well as imaginal exposure to the traumatic memories themselves. These forms of exposure form the basis of PTSD-specific psychotherapies such as prolonged exposure therapy and cognitive processing therapy (Foa, 2011; Resick et al., 2016).

Worksheet 8.1

Identifying Avoidance and Its Consequences

What are your current medical and physical limitations based on medical advice?

Activity, situation, or sensation that is avoided	Distress caused by activity or sensation (0–10)	Short-term consequences of avoiding	Long-term consequences of avoiding	Is the avoidance reasonable based on medical/physical limitations and public health guidelines?	How meaningful or important is the activity or situation? (0–10)

Worksheet 8.2
Engaging in Avoided Activities

Pre-Activity

Goal: What activity do you want to engage in? Why is this important or meaningful to you?

Plan: When, where, and how will you do it?

How distressing do you imagine this activity will be on a 0-to-10 scale?

What barriers do you anticipate getting in the way of your goal?
What can you do to help yourself engage in the situation?
What can you tell yourself?

Post-Activity

How much distress do you feel on a 0-to-10 scale?

What did you learn? How do you feel now?

CHAPTER 9

Module 9: Managing Cognitive Difficulties and "Brain Fog"

Chapter Overview

The purpose of this chapter is to discuss common post-COVID-19 cognitive difficulties and symptoms of brain fog, and their association with the cognitive behavioral model. The content in this chapter will help clients implement behavioral strategies to manage cognitive lapses in daily life. Two worksheets are provided in this module—Worksheet 9.1: Monitoring Cognitive Lapses and Worksheet 9.2: My Cognitive Strategy Plan.

Number of Sessions

The recommended number of sessions is two or three, although more sessions may be required if the client's primary concern is their cognitive difficulties and brain fog symptoms. Consider administering self-report symptom questionnaires (e.g., PHQ-9, GAD-7) at the beginning of the session to continue tracking symptoms of depression and anxiety. Additionally, you may find it helpful to administer a self-report measure of cognitive functioning such as the Patient-Reported Outcomes Measurement Information System (PROMIS) cognitive function scale (Saffer et al., 2015). Finally, if cognitive symptoms appear to be your client's chief complaint, it may be helpful to refer them for a neuro-psychological evaluation if such a service is available to the client and covered by insurance. Such an evaluation can be a helpful roadmap to inform your treatment and consideration of referral to a provider with special expertise in cognitive rehabilitation.

Psychoeducation on COVID-19 and Neurocognitive Function

Cognitive deficits occur in individuals with persisting symptoms of COVID-19. In our own work with hospitalized patients recovering from COVID-19 during the first wave of the pandemic, we observed a high frequency of mild cognitive deficits (Jaywant et al., 2021). COVID-19 tends to affect attention, processing speed, executive functions, and memory. Why these changes occur is still unknown, but they may be due to persistent inflammation, autoimmune activity, or the effect of COVID-19 on the vascular system and blood circulation, all of which can impact brain function.

Many clients benefit from psychoeducation framed from the perspective of the brain, particularly those who tend toward self-criticism, self-blame, and guilt for the symptoms they are experiencing. Helping clients to understand their experience from the perspective of the brain can help to label and externalize what they are experiencing, which can lead to a sense of relief that what the client is experiencing is "real" and not their "fault." However, we caution that such brain-based psychoeducation should always be accompanied by emphasis that brain-related changes are *not* necessarily permanent and do *not* necessarily mean that the client's cognition will get worse over time. One study on COVID-19 showed that the brain changes associated with cognitive deficits improved in the 6 months following COVID-19 (Kas et al., 2021). Further, there is not yet any convincing evidence that COVID-19-related cognitive deficits lead to forms of dementia such as Alzheimer's disease—although this may be a worry of your client. This is an important point to emphasize as clients may worry about the permanence and potential for decline in the future.

Psychoeducation should also include a discussion of the plasticity of the brain—that is, its ability to adapt and change in positive ways. Learning new skills, strategies, and techniques to manage cognitive lapses can induce neuroplastic changes in the brain such as axonal growth and synapse formation. While research on COVID-19 is still in its infancy, the same principles may apply, and we recommend reinforcing the point that the human brain has the capacity to rewire and change in positive ways, even after an illness.

Below is a sample script for how to introduce this session:

> *"For today's session and the next few sessions, I want to focus on how COVID-19 has impacted your cognitive function. By 'cognitive function' I'm referring to cognitive abilities and thinking skills. These are abilities that allow us to efficiently perform our day-to-day activities like working, socializing, and managing our medications and bills. After COVID-19, some people feel as if their thinking is slowed down (we call that slowed processing speed); have difficulty focusing for long periods of time or are easily distracted (we refer to that as attention); have difficulty multitasking; feel overwhelmed by lots of information all at once; and have trouble organizing. Some people describe this as 'brain fog.'*
>
> *We don't yet know exactly why these cognitive difficulties arise in some people after COVID-19, but it may relate to immune activity, inflammation, or changes to our blood circulation and how these factors affect the brain. The good news is that studies suggest that after COVID-19, these difficulties can get better over time. There is no convincing evidence that COVID-19 results in dementia or necessarily means that cognition continues to get worse over time. What we do know from decades of neuroscience research is that the brain has the capacity to adapt by learning new strategies, tools, and ways of doing things. That's what I want us to focus on. But first, I'd like to get a sense of how cognitive difficulties may affect you in your day-to-day life."*

Therapist Note

"Brain fog" is a term that survivors of COVID-19 often use to describe the subjective experience of post-COVID-19 cognitive changes. It typically encompasses the experience of "feeling in a fog," which can be characterized by feeling mentally slowed down, being quick to fatigue mentally, feeling confused or overwhelmed by large amounts of information, and having trouble multitasking. We have found that there are both pros and cons of the use of the term "brain fog." The popularization of the term in the public consciousness during the pandemic has helped to center the experience and narratives of individuals with COVID-19 within the public health and medical communities. On the other hand, "brain fog" is a vague and nonspecific term, which can make it hard to

know what exactly a client is referring to and struggling with and subsequently making it more difficult to tailor cognitive strategies to your client. In this chapter, we use the terms "cognitive difficulties" and "brain fog" interchangeably. If your client has heard of the term "brain fog" and feels that that term best captures what they are experiencing, then it can be helpful to use their language when discussing psychoeducation and treatment. Otherwise, the term "cognitive difficulties" can be sufficient, although we recommend explaining what is meant by "cognition." Even if your client comes to therapy using the term "brain fog," we recommend exploring and probing what your client specifically means by "brain fog" because it can vary from person to person.

Psychoeducation on Cognitive Symptoms and the Cognitive Behavioral Model

There is a bidirectional link between cognitive difficulties and thoughts, emotions, and behaviors. Review the cognitive behavioral model with your client. Point out that cognitive difficulties and symptoms of brain fog can be caused by COVID-19. These cognitive difficulties can result in unhelpful thoughts, distressing emotions, and unhelpful behaviors such as avoidance and reassurance seeking. These thoughts, emotions, and behaviors can exacerbate, amplify, and perpetuate cognitive difficulties. Unhelpful thoughts and distressing emotions in reaction to cognitive challenges can interfere with cognitive processing. Similarly, in response to cognitive challenges, your client may engage in avoidance of cognitively demanding situations. Avoidance prevents learning and practicing strategies to manage cognitive errors. Case Vignette 9.1 highlights these points.

Case Vignette 9.1

THERAPIST: *Can you tell me about some of the difficulties you've been experiencing in thinking, concentrating, and remembering?*

CLIENT: *I feel like I'm really slowed down cognitively. It takes me twice as long to complete a task that would've been a piece of cake before I got COVID.*

THERAPIST: *That sounds tough. What else have you noticed?*

CLIENT: *It's really hard for me to juggle multiple things at the same time, like if my kid is asking me for something and I'm trying to focus on a work call. I just get really overwhelmed, and I can't stay focused. Sometimes it's hard to remember things, too.*

THERAPIST: *I can imagine some of these difficulties have really impacted your life.*

CLIENT: *Yes, it's harder for me to be efficient at work and feel like I'm an equal parent and partner at home. It's frustrating and demoralizing.*

THERAPIST: *I can see how difficult some of these cognitive symptoms have made it for you to live your life. They sound like a real change from before you had COVID. As I mentioned earlier, research suggests that COVID can result in the kinds of cognitive difficulties you're describing. The good news is that there are strategies we can use to help you manage these symptoms and be more efficient and effective in your daily life. Some research even suggests that cognitive difficulties after COVID-19 may improve over time.*

CLIENT: *That makes me feel a little more hopeful.*

THERAPIST: *Let's look at the cognitive behavioral model together to see how our thoughts, emotions, and behavioral responses relate to neurocognitive symptoms* [therapist takes out Worksheet 2.1: Cognitive Behavioral Model, or shares screen with model and worksheet if a telehealth session]. *Notice that cognitive symptoms can result in unhelpful thoughts, distressing emotions, and unhelpful behaviors. You mentioned feeling frustrated earlier—how else have these cognitive difficulties affected your thoughts, emotions, and behaviors?*

CLIENT: *Yeah, I definitely feel frustrated. When I get distracted, I get frustrated at myself. I think, "Why can't you just stay on task?" When I can't remember something, I get pretty anxious. I get in my head a bit and wonder, "Would this have happened before? Why is this happening to me?" I'm having my partner take on more of the childcare responsibilities.*

THERAPIST: *All those thoughts, emotions, and reactions make a lot of sense. Many people with cognitive difficulties after COVID describe thinking and feeling similarly. I'm curious—when these thoughts and emotions come up after a cognitive challenge, does it make it easier or harder to focus or to remember?*

CLIENT: *Oh, harder, for sure. I'm in my head worrying about how things have changed and it's even harder for me to focus.*

THERAPIST: *That's a very common pattern. Often anxious or self-critical thoughts or heightened emotions can worsen cognitive difficulties* [therapist points to CBT model showing how thoughts/emotions/behaviors loop back to affect neurocognitive symptoms]. *Our mental processing capacity is a finite resource, and when some of that mental processing goes toward thinking about the past or the future or is caught up in unhelpful thoughts or difficult emotions, it makes it even harder to focus or remember things. A useful analogy is that we all have a mental "blackboard." That "blackboard" is responsible for holding on to the information we need at any given time to focus, remember, solve problems, and efficiently manage ongoing cognitive demands. When space on that blackboard is taken up by thoughts and emotions, it's harder for our brains to think, focus, and remember.*

CLIENT: *OK, that makes sense. But what do I do about that?*

THERAPIST: *Good question. What this means is that we need to implement cognitive strategies to help you focus, remember, multitask, and be more efficient. But we also need to implement strategies to help you manage unhelpful thoughts and distressing emotions when cognitive difficulties come up, so that you're not inadvertently making it harder on yourself. We also want to watch out for avoidance, because that'll limit the opportunities you have to practice the skills and strategies. But before we learn strategies, let's get a better understanding of your difficulties in thinking and what factors affect these difficulties.*

Monitoring Cognitive Lapses

As a first step, prior to discussing and implementing cognitive strategies, introduce and assign for homework Worksheet 9.1: Monitoring Cognitive Lapses. Worksheets can be found at the end of this chapter in both the Therapist Guide and Client Workbook or can be accessed by searching for this book's title on the Oxford Academic platform, at academic.oup.com.

The purpose of this worksheet is to start to have the client self-monitor and increase their awareness of cognitive lapses that occur in daily life; associated thoughts, emotions, and behaviors; and any strategies or systems that are being attempted to try and manage the cognitive difficulty. It can be helpful to fill out an example in session using the client's retrospective recall of an event over the past week. Then assign Worksheet 9.1 for homework, with the client logging cognitive lapses that occur throughout the week. The easiest way for a client to do this is to have the worksheet available in a central location and write down instances as they happen. Alternatively, the client can fill it out as a diary at the end of the day. You may need to problem-solve ways to help the client remember to use the worksheet. Involving a trusted caregiver can be helpful.

Cognitive Strategies

The second session should start with a review of Worksheet 9.1. This will start to give you an idea of the types of lapses that are occurring; the environmental and situational factors affecting these events; the client's thoughts, emotions, and behaviors; and the type of strategies and systems the client may have tried to implement already. Next, use the following framework in session to develop a plan to implement cognitive strategies. This can be completed using Worksheet 9.2: My Cognitive Strategy Plan, which can be found at the end of this chapter in both the Therapist Guide and Client Workbook or can be accessed by searching for this book's title on the Oxford Academic platform, at academic.oup.com.

Step 1: Set a Goal

Collaboratively work with your client to set a specific, actionable, realistic goal related to improving cognitive function. Perhaps your client's goal is to be able to sustain their attention on a work task for 30 minutes at a time. Or your client may want to remember to take their medication consistently without missing a dosage.

Step 2: Decide on a Strategy or System

This is where Socratic questioning and problem-solving comes in. Start with general, open-ended questions about how the client may have previously tried to manage a cognitive difficulty. Worksheet 9.1 can be helpful here as a launching point for discussion. Probe for modifications to existing strategies. It can be more effective to build on strategies and systems the client already has in place than to start from scratch. The following are example questions that can be used to probe strategies and systems the client may have attempted (Toglia & Foster, 2021):

> *"I want to get a sense of how you've tried to manage [cognitive difficulty]. What strategies, methods, or system have you tried to help?"*

Next, try to probe for how these existing strategies or systems could be modified, or how new strategies could be adopted. This step is akin to the classic problem-solving strategy in cognitive-behavioral therapy where the therapist helps the client generate a list of solutions to a problem and reflect on the pros/benefits and cons/costs before choosing and trying out a solution.

"What do you think you could do differently? What strategy, system, or method might help you work through this cognitive challenge?"

If the client can self-generate novel, alternate, or modified strategies, then proceed to asking them about the pros and cons and exploring whether this possible strategy makes sense to implement. Commonly, clients may say, "I'm not sure what I can do" or turn it back to you as the therapist, saying, "What do you think I should do?" In these cases, and to generate ideas, refer to the "List of Cognitive Strategies" below.

Step 3: Create a Plan to Implement the Cognitive Strategy or System

Ask the client the following questions to help create a plan to implement a cognitive strategy:

- When, and in what situations, will the strategy be implemented?
- Do any materials (e.g., a notebook) need to be acquired beforehand?
- What are some barriers that are anticipated and how can they be addressed proactively?
- How will the client remember to use the strategy ("remember to remember")? This may necessitate the use of a strategically placed reminder, such as on the client's desk or a smartphone alert. Involving a family member, spouse, caregiver, or housemate in this discussion can be key as this person can help to provide reminders and to increase motivation.

After a week of implementing the agreed-upon strategy, review with your client at the following session how it went. Often, modifications may be required, and trouble-shooting may be needed to overcome barriers and issues. Use a new copy of Worksheet 9.2 to rewrite the plan for the upcoming week and subsequent weeks.

List of Cognitive Strategies

Many of these strategies are adapted from existing approaches and workbooks for attention-deficit/hyperactivity disorder (Safren et al., 2017), traumatic brain injury (Twamley et al., 2010), and neurologic illness more broadly (Toglia et al., 2012). We recommend that you refer to these workbooks, manuals, and papers for additional strategies that can be helpful for your client.

1. **Write important information down.** Writing information down in a notepad/notebook or on a smartphone "notes" app means the information is better attended to and available for later reference. Problem-solve with your client where they may write information down (a small pocket-sized book, a planner, on a document on their smartphone) and in what circumstances they will write information down. Examples of information that can benefit from being written down includes auditory information that needs to be remembered and/or acted on later, an important detail from a conversation, a request from a work colleague, or even the name of an individual the client has just met.

2. **Create a task list, prioritize, and check tasks off.** To help your client organize their tasks, suggest that they write a task list either each morning or the night before. They should rate the tasks based on their importance. For example, the tasks that need to be completed that day are assigned a high priority and are the first ones slotted into the client's daily schedule when planning the day. Those tasks with a medium priority are scheduled into the day only after the high-priority tasks are scheduled. Low-priority tasks are those that don't need to be completed that day, even though the client would like to keep them on their list for eventual completion. Tasks should also be scheduled in such a way that they are appropriately paced to minimize fatigue (see Chapter 10 for further details).

3. **Break tasks up into smaller, individual subtasks.** Large tasks and projects can feel overwhelming to clients. Thus, it is helpful to collaborate with your client to take individual tasks—likely ones that the client is struggling to make headway on—and break them into smaller subtasks. The smaller subtasks are then put individually into daily task lists and schedules.

4. **Make environmental modifications.** For clients who struggle with distractions, discuss and problem-solve ways in which the environment can be modified to better focus and enhance cognitive efficiency and task completion by mitigating distractions. Examples include closing the door or moving to a quiet room when working (auditory distractions) and closing window blinds (visual distractions). The client can also modify the immediate environment to eliminate distractions, for example by closing tabs on a web browser or deleting/hiding social media apps on a smartphone.

5. **Use technological aids.** Technology, particularly smartphones and associated applications, can facilitate cognitive performance. Spend time exploring with your client how they use their smartphone and what factors might be helpful and which might be barriers to effective cognitive function. Many clients prefer using a calendar application on their phone to manage appointments.

6. **Do a verbal rehearsal.** Using "self-talk" (also referred to as "verbal rehearsal") can be a helpful strategy for some clients, for example those who describe short-term memory lapses akin to "I walked into a room and couldn't remember what I needed" or "I walked into the grocery store and couldn't remember what I wanted to buy." Mentally rehearsing the information they need to remember keeps it active in working memory (the mental blackboard) and prevents it from being forgotten.

7. **Use visualization.** Visualization is a powerful strategy that can be paired with verbal rehearsal. Suggest that the client visualize in their mind's eye the information they need to remember or the future intention they hope to remember and execute. Visualization strengthens the information in memory and can make it more likely that the client will recall the action to initiate at the time or event that it is intended.

Therapist Note

Many clients struggle with the notion of using cognitive strategies because they perceive these techniques as "crutches." The use of cognitive strategies may elicit negative self-appraisals and beliefs. These include thoughts such as "I should be able to do this on my own" or "I didn't have to do this before. Why should I have to do it now?" Another thought that often comes up is "Well, if I use this strategy, aren't I just 'covering' for this deficit rather than actively working to improve it?" We recommend empathically normalizing these responses and providing the following psychoeducation:

1. *Normalize the use of strategies. The reality is that we all use strategies, but often we do it automatically without consciously thinking about it. Putting appointments in a Google calendar, writing a grocery list on a sticky note, and taking notes on a lecture in class are all strategies. Depending on your comfort with self-disclosure, and your conceptualization of how self-disclosure might be perceived by the client, it can be helpful to provide an example of a strategy you yourself might use in your daily life. A common one for many therapists is taking session notes to keep track of, and remember, session content from week to week.*

2. *We also often need to adapt and modify the strategies we use to fit evolving situations and circumstances. That's what managing post-COVID-19 cognitive difficulties entails: managing tasks and information in different ways than what we were used to. While beforehand many strategies may have been automatic and unconscious, now they must be more conscious and intentionally implemented. The more a new strategy is practiced, the more routine and effortless it will become.*

3. *Research has shown that the use of cognitive strategies is associated with changes in the brain. Thus, using cognitive strategies might actually change the brain and is not just "covering" for a deficit as a crutch.*

Managing Thoughts, Emotions, and Behaviors Arising from Cognitive Difficulties

As noted earlier in this chapter, how your client responds to a cognitive lapse, error, or challenge—specifically their thoughts, emotions, and behaviors—can exacerbate, amplify, and perpetuate cognitive difficulties and symptoms of brain fog. Collaborate with the client to discuss unhelpful thoughts in relation to cognitive difficulties. Help the client to reframe any unhelpful thoughts and to self-generate thoughts that are more helpful, motivating, and self-compassionate. An adaptive thought acknowledges that a cognitive lapse has occurred but "turns the temperature down" on the client's tendency to self-blame, overgeneralize, or catastrophize. Example prompts to elicit such helpful thoughts include:

- *"What's something you can tell yourself when [specific cognitive lapse] happens that is more helpful and present-focused?"*
- *"What's something you can tell yourself when [specific cognitive lapse] happens that is kind to yourself and acknowledges the difficulty of the situation without blaming yourself?"*

Helpful thoughts might include:

- *"I didn't remember what I needed to, but I'm learning new tools and techniques to improve. It takes time."*
- *"It's OK to get distracted sometimes! Not everybody can stay focused 100% of the time."*
- *"Having trouble remembering a name now doesn't mean it will always be this way. I'm doing my best."*

Note any unhelpful behaviors your client is engaging in. Your client may avoid cognitively demanding activities out of fear of experiencing a cognitive lapse. Avoidance typically worsens mood, limits function, and limits opportunities to implement cognitive strategies. Another maladaptive behavior to assess for and mitigate is excessive checking and rumination. In response to a cognitive lapse, your client may engage in actively thinking about all the recent instances in which they became distracted or could not remember a piece of information. They may actively ruminate about all the ways in which their cognition is different from how they were functioning prior to contracting COVID-19. If they are uncertain about whether a certain cognitive lapse would have occurred prior to COVID-19, then they may search for an "answer" to resolve this uncertainty—for example, by seeking reassurance from a spouse, family member, or friend. Although some self-reflection can help to promote awareness and behavioral change, excessively worrying and reassurance-seeking takes up important cognitive resources on the mental "blackboard" and makes it even less likely that your client will be able to focus or remember.

To increase awareness of the impact of these behaviors and to help develop more adaptive behaviors, ask your client whether avoiding, excessively focusing/ruminating, or reassurance-seeking results in better or worse cognitive function in the short term and long term. Does it make it more likely or not that the client will experience a cognitive lapse? The function of these behaviors is typically to reduce distress or to establish a sense of control in the short term. Unfortunately, these behaviors can worsen mood, anxiety, and neurocognitive function in the long term.

To counteract avoidance tendencies, encourage the client to approach situations that may elicit cognitive lapses. The way these situations are approached may be different from before the client contracted COVID-19. That is, the client should approach these situations in ways that incorporate cognitive strategies (see above) and create a likelihood for success. It may mean reducing the cognitive load of activities by asking for help, shortening a task, pacing activities, or breaking a task up into subtasks—but the client should typically not try to avoid tasks entirely in response to negative thoughts and emotions about the situation.

To mitigate a tendency for worry, rumination, or reassurance-seeking, it can be helpful to promote present-moment focus. This can also be helpful for the emotions that inevitably arise during a cognitive lapse—emotions such as anxiety, fear, anger, frustration, and sadness. Refer to the techniques in Chapter 5 on mindfulness to help your client stay present-focused. Any of the tools and techniques related to mindfulness and self-compassion can be helpful here. Simple diaphragmatic breathing or five-finger breathing can help ground your client in the moment; prevent rumination, worry, or reassurance-seeking; and make it more likely they will be able to sustain focus or retrieve the information from memory that is sought after.

At-Home Practice

Remind the client that out-of-session practice of the skills learned in this chapter is crucial for the client to see changes in their symptoms over time. In the first session, assign Worksheet 9.1 for at-home practice. In the second and subsequent sessions, assign Worksheet 9.2. The plan that is developed using Worksheet 9.2 can be refined and revised over time.

Worksheet 9.1
Monitoring Cognitive Lapses

Think of a recent time when you had a "lapse" in your thinking—was it hard for you to find the right word? Did you struggle to multi-task? Become distracted? Have a hard time processing information? Write down your experience in the table below:

(1) Situation	(2) What happened?	(3) What thoughts did you have in response?	(4) What emotions did you experience?	(5) What did you do in response?	(6) Other possible contributing factors?

Worksheet 9.2
My Cognitive Strategy Plan

Goal

- What specific, actionable, and realistic cognitively-based goal do I want to work towards?

My Strategy

- What systems already in place can I modify?
- How can I break the task down into subtasks?
- Could I use one of the following strategies:
  - *Write information down*
  - *Create and use a checklist*
  - *Modify the environment*
  - *Use technology*
  - *Use self-talk*
  - *Use visualization*

Implementation

- When will I implement the strategy?
- Do I need to acquire materials beforehand?
- How will I remember to implement the plan?
- What might get in the way?

CHAPTER 10

Module 10: Fatigue and Sleep

Chapter Overview

The purpose of this chapter is to discuss fatigue and sleep disturbances as sequelae of COVID-19 and to help your client implement behavioral strategies to manage fatigue and improve sleep. Two worksheets are provided in this chapter—Worksheet 10.1: Rating Activities and Fatigue and Worksheet 10.2: Activity Pacing.

Number of Sessions

Two or three sessions are recommended for this chapter. Consider administering self-report symptom questionnaires (e.g., PHQ-9, GAD-7) at the beginning of the session to continue tracking symptoms of depression and anxiety. Additionally, you may find it helpful to administer a self-report measure of cognitive functioning such as the PROMIS fatigue scale (Ameringer et al., 2016) and/or the PROMIS sleep disturbance and sleep-related impairment scales (Yu et al., 2012).

Therapeutic Content

Psychoeducation on COVID-19 and Fatigue

Fatigue is common and debilitating after COVID-19. Like many of the persisting effects of COVID-19, we do not yet know what causes fatigue. It may be a similar mechanism to lingering physical and cognitive symptoms. Nevertheless, fatigue can be managed, and you can have an impactful role in helping clients manage their fatigue.

Cognitive behavioral techniques can help clients to better manage fatigue (though like other sequelae of COVID-19, it is not intended to "cure" fatigue). Learning to develop healthier activity patterns, reframe thoughts, and use mindfulness techniques to decrease overfocus on symptoms can be powerful tools to manage fatigue. The techniques described here are adapted from CBT protocols (Gotaas et al., 2021; Starbuck et al., 2022) and from our own clinical experience working with clients with COVID-19 experiencing fatigue. In the context of the cognitive behavioral model of COVID-19, fatigue can be conceptualized as a physical symptom that impacts, and is impacted by, a client's thoughts, emotions, and behaviors.

Therapist Note

Many of the strategies below are tailored for individuals with persistent, chronic fatigue. The relationship between fatigue and thoughts, emotions, and behaviors can be conceptualized somewhat differently for clients with acute fatigue, for example those who are hospitalized, were just discharged from the hospital, and/or are in an acute recovery period from illness. In that context, fatigue can be thought of as a "true alarm"—a signal to reduce activity as the body channels energy toward recovery and slowly rebuilds its energy capacity. Thus, when working with clients who are still in the hospital or are just past the acute period of COVID-19 infectious symptoms, we have found that validating the experience of fatigue as a normal and adaptive phenomenon is paramount. Strategies for pacing activities and graded activity increase can still be helpful, however.

For many COVID-19 clients without a history of chronic medical, physical, or psychiatric illness, fatigue is a new and difficult challenge to navigate. Often, clients engage in behavioral responses to attempt to control or mitigate fatigue that can be (temporarily) helpful in the short term but perpetuate fatigue in the long term. Introduce and discuss the following maladaptive long-term strategies to control fatigue. Emphasize the difference between the short-term effects of the behavior (which can typically be temporarily positive and reinforcing) and the long-term effects of the behavior (which are typically unhelpful and maladaptive).

1. **Under-exertion:** A natural reaction to feelings of tiredness and exhaustion is to think that the body needs rest, and that one should

restrict or stop activity. Fatigue is at times an important signal to rest, particularly for clients who have recently recovered from COVID-19 or who were recently hospitalized. In contrast, overreacting to chronic fatigue by significantly cutting back on activities can have negative long-term impacts. Chronic under-exertion or underactivity can worsen fatigue. It can fuel a belief that activity is dangerous or intolerable. Further, non-use of muscles can lead to weakening and atrophy that physiologically decreases activity tolerance and increases fatigue even further. Under-exertion and diminished activity can also worsen mood and symptoms of depression.

2. **Over-exertion:** Fatigue can be highly variable after COVID-19. This results in "good days" and "bad days." Trying to fit as much activity into a good day or good period is an understandable and common reaction with a long-term negative impact. Over-exertion can bring on several days' worth of fatigue. Many times, the fatigue signal does not kick in until after the client has over-exerted themselves, at which point it is too late to reduce activity. This is often referred to in the literature as the "boom and bust" cycle.

3. **Excessive focus on the body's energy level:** A theme in these behavioral responses is a tendency to react abruptly to situational and fluctuating feelings of fatigue. Sometimes, as a precursor to a feeling of impending fatigue or "crash," clients may spend excessive time checking in on physical sensations and their current fatigue level. They may try to gauge their fatigue and to compare their energy level to how they felt the day before, the week before, or even prior to contracting COVID-19. While some self-monitoring is important to implement adaptive behavioral strategies (see below), excessive focus on the body's energy state can result in a tendency to overreact to normal fluctuations in energy level.

After introducing these maladaptive behavioral responses to fatigue, lead the client in a discussion of how some of these behaviors may manifest in their own life. Ask how your client typically responds to feeling fatigued, whether they have reduced their activity level over time or have overexerted themselves or "overdone it" at times. You can also probe as to the frequency and intensity of focus on fatigue signals in their body. If your client keeps a calendar or schedule, and particularly if it is electronic, it can be helpful to incorporate this in the chapter. Try and maintain a compassionate and validating stance throughout this discussion, noting that these behaviors are all *completely understandable* given the client's experience—there just may be more helpful ways of responding to fatigue than what the client has done to date.

Unhelpful Thoughts in the Context of Fatigue

A client's thoughts, beliefs, and appraisals about fatigue can also perpetuate and intensify the experience of fatigue. Engaging in repetitive negative or unhelpful thinking can be exhausting in and of itself, which adds to the sense of fatigue. In the context of the cognitive behavioral model, thoughts and beliefs about fatigue can also lead to under- or over-exertion. Probe the client for their own unique thoughts, beliefs, and appraisals about fatigue. The following thoughts, beliefs, and appraisals about fatigue can occur:

- *"I'm always going to feel tired."*
- *"I'll never be the same as I was before I got sick."*
- *"If I engage in any activity, it's just going to make the fatigue worse."*
- *"There's something wrong with me that I can't even tolerate [simple activity]."*
- *"I should feel energized and be able to manage my responsibilities."*

You can also use the above sample thoughts to ask the client, "Do you have similar thoughts?" In our experience, clients recovering from COVID-19—particularly those who were previously in good physical health—may have core beliefs related to activity. It may therefore be helpful to explore fatigue in terms of what it means for their sense of self and personal identity. Further exploration of how to manage unhelpful thoughts and beliefs is presented in Chapter 7: Reframing Unhelpful Thoughts.

Behavioral Strategies to Manage Fatigue

Behavioral strategies to manage fatigue are complementary and interwoven and involve planning and modifying activities to (1) gauge energy output and maintain a relatively consistent output; (2) plan activity schedules ahead of time so that energy-intensive activities are scheduled at times when energy is likely to be higher; and (3) intersperse breaks and pace activities. These strategies are adapted from treatments for chronic illness, chronic pain, and chronic fatigue.

Gauging Energy Expenditure and Fatigue

A helpful way to begin discussion of the client's daily energy expenditure and fatigue is to make it experiential; anchor the discussion around the client's own schedule in session. If the client uses an electronic calendar, then encourage them to share it in session. At this point, it can be helpful to look at the client's schedule for the past week and the upcoming week. The schedule will likely include appointments or other one-time events; however, it is also important to explore routine activities that the client engages in but may not make it onto the calendar. Such routine tasks can include dressing, bathing, meal preparation, cooking, childcare, driving to/from work, and other work-related tasks. You may start to notice the following patterns:

- A busy schedule with many back-to-back activities. This can be a clue to overexertion.
- A relative paucity of activities throughout the week. This may suggest that the client has decreased their activity output and is underexerting themselves.
- Variability and inconsistency in activity durations, both within a day and across several days. For example, a client may have several activities planned in succession on a given morning, with nothing planned in the afternoon or evening because they anticipate feeling fatigued. Or the client may have a heavy activity schedule early in the week with minimal activity on the weekend. These activity patterns can be markers of the boom/bust cycle.

Once you have a good sense of the client's week and how activities with different energy expenditures are typically spread over the week, the goal is to plan and pace activities strategically to balance energy output. Work collaboratively with the client—in session—to plan activities for the following week. Use Worksheet 10.1: Rating Activities and Fatigue to make a list of the client's activities for the coming week and help them determine how fatiguing they anticipate the activities may be. Worksheets can be found at the end of this chapter in both the Therapist Guide and Client Workbook or can be accessed by searching for this book's title on the Oxford Academic platform, at academic.oup.com. Using the ratings from Worksheet 10.1, work collaboratively with your client to help them schedule activities over the next week that manage the amount of energy expended. Activities should be balanced so that activities that require high energy and are highly fatiguing are interspersed throughout the week, as are those that require moderate energy and are moderately fatiguing. The goal is to keep the overall energy output *feasible* given the client's fatigue level and generally *consistent* day by day.

When planning the schedule, activities that are moderately to highly fatiguing and have flexibility in scheduling should be scheduled for optimal-energy times. Explain to the client that they should avoid bunching or grouping highly fatiguing activities all together because this can result in a common but maladaptive strategy where the client attempts to "do it all at once while I'm feeling good." As part of planning activities, encourage the client to break lengthy activities that require high energy levels and are highly fatiguing into subtasks or smaller components spread throughout the week.

Finally, many clients also have activities in their lives that they find restorative, energizing, or reinvigorating. That is, they may feel *more* energy after engaging in such activities. Explore with your client the possible presence of restorative or reinvigorating activities and encourage them to schedule such activities throughout the week.

Pacing Activities

Another key component of managing fatigue is interspersing activities with breaks and periods of rest and respite. This is referred to as "activity pacing." Using Worksheet 10.2: Activity Pacing in session with the client, list the client's planned activities for the week with a focus on those that require moderate or high energy expenditure. Then work with the client to plan the amount of time that will be spent on the activity ("planned goal time") before a rest of specified duration is taken ("planned rest time"). During the week, the client will log how long they actually spend on the activity as well as the actual time they spend resting afterwards. They will also rate their fatigue level afterwards as well as any accompanying thoughts and emotions. A critical concept to impart to the client is that they should engage in energy-demanding and fatiguing tasks for a shorter period than they initially think they can, schedule a break earlier than they would normally plan, and take a break of longer duration than they would normally think to take. This is because we often overestimate how much we can really do without becoming fatigued. Thus, if a client thinks they can work for 20 minutes on a task before taking a break, encourage them to try working for 15 minutes instead.

For clients with more moderate to severe overall fatigue based on your assessment, breaks and periods of rest should be relatively long (i.e., 30 minutes, 1 hour). For clients with mild fatigue, particularly those who are working and have demanding schedules, encourage them to include brief breaks and periods of respite throughout the day (e.g., leaving a 5-minute gap in between Zoom meetings).

After the goal times and rest times are set on Worksheet 10.2, then this information can be used to further modify the client's weekly schedule to help them structure their activity schedule. Activities should be scheduled for the lengths that were decided on and breaks should also be scheduled for the duration agreed upon. Importantly, breaks should be explicitly scheduled into the client's calendar as "events" to mitigate a tendency to overwork or to mindlessly keep working on tasks.

Therapist Note

The therapy session is a good time to model pacing and taking breaks. Ask your client how long they can attend and engage during a session before their attention begins to drift. Inquire as to whether they feel fatigued after a typical 45- to 50-minute therapy hour. Depending on how long you've been working with the client, you may already have a good sense of this through your clinical observations. Use this information to build in brief breaks during your session.

Sometimes clients are resistant to the idea of pacing activities on good days when they are feeling minimal fatigue. Underlying this resistance can be a desire to be as efficient as possible—as efficient as they were before COVID-19—and the thought that they will fall further behind if they do not capitalize on as many "good" hours as they have. In these situations, it is helpful to acknowledge and validate the client's thoughts and feelings reflecting a desire to return to doing things the way they could have before COVID-19. Further, it is helpful to explore the short-term benefit versus the long-term cost of the strategy of cramming as much as possible into good days. Has this worked for the client in the past? Is this the most efficient *in the long term*? Highlight that even though pacing means including more frequent/longer breaks, it typically *increases* efficiency and work output in the long run.

Mitigating Overfocus on Fatigue and Physical Symptoms

For clients who tend to be excessively focused on and vigilant about fatigue, it can be helpful to incorporate relaxation and mindfulness exercises that encourage awareness of body sensations and subsequently shift the focus of attention to the external environment. If you have already completed Chapters 5 and 6 (mindfulness and relaxation), those exercises can be reviewed and implemented in the setting of fatigue. Diaphragmatic breathing and imagery may be helpful here. To shift the focus of attention to the external environment, use the mindfulness-based exercise shown in Box 10.1 in session to expand awareness of the environment via sensory experience.

Box 10.1 5-4-3-2-1 Mindfulness Exercise

Gently bring your awareness to your breath. Start to slow your breathing so you become aware of each in-breath and each out-breath.

Bring your attention to the environment around you. Notice five things that you see around you. With each breath, shift your attention to something else that you see in the environment.

Now, notice four sounds that you hear in the environment around you. With each breath, shift your attention to something else that you hear.

Next, notice three things that you feel. It could be the feeling of floor on your feet, your back against a chair, or the clothes against your body. With each breath, shift your attention to something else that you feel.

Then, notice two things that you smell. With each breath, shift your attention to something else that you smell.

And finally, take one more breath and notice any taste in your mouth and on your tongue.

Strategies to Manage Sleep Disruption

Sleep disruption can occur after COVID-19. Below, we describe strategies to facilitate sleep initiation and sleep maintenance. Note that these strategies are adapted from resources such as the American Academy of Sleep Medicine and implemented based on our experience working with clients with COVID-19. Many of these strategies fall under the umbrella term "sleep hygiene." If your client has significant and severe sleep disruption that you conceptualize as the primary symptom impacting function, we recommend considering implementing a sleep-focused intervention such as Cognitive Behavioral Therapy for Insomnia (CBT-I). If your client's sleep disturbance is related to a primary diagnosis of post-traumatic stress disorder (PTSD), then using an intervention specific for PTSD may be indicated. There are also targeted treatments specifically for the experience of nightmares. For clients whose sleep difficulties are one component of the constellation of their symptoms, the following techniques can help, many of which integrate skills introduced in other chapters.

Pre-Sleep Routine

Preparing the body for sleep often requires planning a "wind-down" routine several hours prior to sleep initiation. It also requires implementing behaviors that prepare the mind and body for sleep. Explore your client's typical afternoon, evening, and nighttime behaviors and activities. For example:

- What do the afternoon and evening typically look like for your client?
- Is your client engaging in highly stimulating activities and then abruptly attempting to go to sleep?
- How late in the day does your client consume caffeine, if any?
- Does the client typically drink alcoholic beverages in the evening?
- Is the client staying up late purposefully?

All the above behaviors can interfere with sleep.

Problem-solve with your client how to modify these behaviors, should they exist and be interfering with sleep. Oftentimes maladaptive sleep-promoting behaviors are automatic and routine; the client is likely to engage in them without even realizing. Having a plan can help break the client out of being on "autopilot." Clients with post-COVID-19 neurocognitive difficulties may also forget to implement novel and adaptive sleep-promoting behaviors. Involving a spouse, caregiver, or other family member who lives with the client can be helpful here.

In addition to the above behaviors to eliminate, discuss behaviors to add to the pre-sleep routine to promote a state of relaxation and slowly wind the body down toward rest. Helpful behaviors to add include exercising earlier in the day; scheduling an evening mindfulness practice or relaxation practice; taking a relaxing bath or shower; putting on soothing music or ambient sounds; and engaging in light reading or television watching—but avoid reading or watching highly evocative, emotional, or stimulating content.

Sleep Initiation

Your client may have difficulty initiating sleep. Some individuals with persistent sequelae of COVID-19 can experience an increase in worry or ruminative thoughts at nighttime. Without the distractions of daytime activities, work, and social or familial demands, clients may experience their thoughts and emotions as more intense. Upon attempting to fall asleep, clients may experience a heightening of worry and fear about persisting COVID-19 symptoms and their uncertainty, or rumination about experiences during the acute illness phase of COVID-19. Clients may become increasingly aware of and vigilant about physical symptoms—discomfort, weakness, numbness, shortness of breath, and other residual symptoms of COVID-19. If physical symptoms are prominent and interfere with sleep, we recommend the use of relaxation strategies and mindfulness exercises. Using relaxation strategies prior to sleep can help to regulate the fight-or-flight system, decrease sympathetic nervous system activity, and increase parasympathetic nervous system activity.

Environmental modification can also be helpful. Keeping the temperature in the room relatively cool can promote sleep. Using light-blocking shades or a sleep mask can promote darkness that is conducive to sleep.

Closing a door, using white noise, or wearing earplugs can eliminate sounds and distractions that interfere with sleep initiation.

We have found that clients who have been hospitalized in the past may fear and avoid going to sleep. They may fear losing their breath, or even dying, and not being able to do anything about it because they are asleep. They may associate being in bed with distress, fear, pain, and other negative emotions because sleep initiation triggers memories of being in their hospital bed. If fear and avoidance are contributing to poor sleep initiation, we recommend spending time empathically exploring this fear. Validate that the client's experience of fear and desire to avoid sleep is an understandable response—the brain is trying to alert the client to threat, a signal likely triggered by the experience of contracting COVID-19.

Gently review exposure principles and the importance of confronting feared and avoided situations (Chapter 8). While the brain's threat response to sleep may have been a "true alarm" during the initial acute stage of COVID-19, it is more likely that now this response has become a "false alarm"—trying to alert the client to a threat that is no longer present. The more that sleep is avoided, the more the brain will interpret sleep as a dangerous situation and as an ongoing threat. To counteract this, through engaging in sleep, the brain will slowly learn that it does not need to fear sleep. Here, it can also be helpful to go back to Chapter 7: Reframing Unhelpful Thoughts. Work with the client to identify thoughts that may come up when attempting to initiate sleep and develop more helpful, adaptive thoughts.

Sleep Maintenance

Clients may experience nighttime awakenings or interrupted sleep. Sometimes this can happen out of the blue. Clients may wake up from a nightmare, or otherwise feel distressed because being in bed reminds them of a past hospitalization. For a client who wakes up after a nightmare or otherwise feels distressed or hyper-aroused, we recommend a relaxation exercise such as Five-Finger Breathing to counteract elevated sympathetic nervous system activity. If clients cannot reinitiate sleep within approximately 20 to 30 minutes, it can be helpful to listen to gentle music or something mundane like a quiet podcast in a separate room, so that the bedroom does not become associated with wakefulness, distress, or frustration. After about 20 to 30 minutes, the client can return to bed and attempt to re-initiate sleep.

Encourage clients to maintain a consistent wake time, regardless of the amount of time slept, and regardless of whether it's a weekday or weekend. This will help normalize and regularize the sleep–wake cycle. Even if the client has had a poor night's sleep, keeping a consistent wake time is helpful.

At-Home Practice

Explain to the client that, like with learning anything new, practice is essential. Review the importance of out-of-session practice at home. Without practice, the strategies are difficult to engage when they're needed most. With practice, however, the skills will become more effective and more automatic and can be used anytime, anywhere, and with very little effort. This is especially true for strategies to manage fatigue and sleep because many of the activity patterns that contribute to ongoing fatigue and sleep disruption are automatic and routine. Breaking those automatic activity patterns requires conscious effort and deliberate practice over time.

Worksheet 10.1
Rating Activities and Fatigue

Instructions: List routine and non-routine activities that you plan on doing over the next week. Note how often you typically spend on the activity. Rate how fatiguing you anticipate the activity to be. This worksheet will help you schedule these activities strategically so you're balancing your energy output every day and not over- or under-exerting yourself.

Routine Activities

Activity	Time Typically Spent on Activity	Rate Fatigue on 0–10 Scale (Lowest to Highest)

Non-Routine Activities

Activity	Time You Anticipate Spending on Activity	Rate Anticipated Fatigue on 0–10 Scale (Lowest to Highest)

Worksheet 10.2
Activity Pacing

Fatiguing Activity	Planned Goal Time	Planned Rest Time	Actual Time Spent	Actual Time Rested	Fatigue Level Afterwards (0–10)	Thoughts	Emotions

CHAPTER 11

Module 11: Participating In Medical Treatment

Chapter Overview

Medical adherence is essential to clients' well-being and recovery post-COVID-19. The aim of this chapter is to provide strategies to enhance adherence to maximize clients' participation in medical care. The chapter incorporates strategies discussed in pres skill-building chapters to enhance motivation, improve adherence, and address common barriers to treatment engagement. Two worksheets are provided in this chapter—Worksheet 11.1: My Current Medical Care and Worksheet 11.2: Appointment Preparation Form.

Number of Sessions

One or two sessions are recommended for this chapter. Consider administering self-report symptom questionnaires (e.g., PHQ-9, GAD-7) at the beginning of the session to continue tracking symptoms of depression and anxiety.

Therapeutic Content

Adherence as a Therapeutic Target

Poor adherence to medical and rehabilitative recommendations can worsen physical health, lead to disability and impaired functioning, and exacerbate anxiety and mood symptoms. In contrast, increasing adherence can improve daily functioning, reduce disability, and help clients return to a more independent and satisfying life. There is also a reciprocal relationship between adherence and mood. Successful adherence can increase clients' sense of competence and self-efficacy, with beneficial effects on mood and subsequent improvement in treatment engagement.

However, adhering to medical recommendations can be a complex and challenging process for clients with persisting symptoms of COVID-19. Multiple barriers can make it difficult for clients to adhere to medical follow-ups, travel to treatment centers, or pursue a regular physical or occupational therapy program. The strategies introduced in this chapter are intended to increase motivation and adherence to medical treatments. These techniques combine principles from empirically supported interventions designed to improve mood and medical adherence in populations with complex medical illnesses (Alexopoulos et al., 2012, 2018). This chapter also integrates strategies from Motivational Interviewing, which has been shown to increase medical adherence (Martins et al., 2009; Miller & Rollnick, 2012; Palacio et al., 2016). The overall aim is to improve adherence by fostering motivation and establishing personalized strategies to address client-specific barriers to treatment engagement.

Reviewing the Client's Medical Care and Goals

At this point in treatment, you should have a good working knowledge of the client's medical care. This information will have been gathered in part through your initial intake assessment and in part from your therapy sessions, where you may learn about ongoing medical symptoms and how they are being treated over time. Ideally, you will have spoken to your client's medical providers. However, this is a good time to revisit the client's current medical care, and specifically note areas of poor adherence or any difficulties the client has had with engaging in their medical care. It can also be helpful to revisit the tools and techniques from Chapter 1: Setting Goals for Therapy to help the client select a few initial goals related to their medical care. Identifying specific goals can increase adherence to medical care by highlighting the client's desire for change and by serving as reminders to motivate behavior during moments of ambivalence. Goals should be specific, realistic, concrete, measurable, and achievable—for example, *"I want to take my medication daily and only miss at most one dose a week"* or *"I want to participate in physical therapy home exercises three times a week for 1 month."*

Identifying and Troubleshooting Barriers to Adherence

Multiple problems can interfere with adherence to medical and rehabilitation recommendations. Common barriers to treatment engagement among medically complex populations with mood symptoms and anxiety include low motivation or ambivalence about change, psychiatric symptoms (anxiety, depression, poor emotion regulation), practical barriers to accessing treatment, cognitive difficulties, misconceptions about COVID-19 and its medical symptoms and treatment, dissatisfaction with treatment, and cultural factors, including mistrust of healthcare systems due to pervasive, systemic racism.

The reasons for poor adherence may be numerous and vary widely from client to client. This diversity in barriers requires a personalized approach. Your aim is to identify client-specific barriers and help develop concrete strategies to address them, with the goal of maximizing medical treatment adherence and medical outcomes. In the sections below, we describe approaches to assess each barrier and corresponding interventions to overcome them. Worksheets can be found at the end of this chapter in both the Therapist Guide and Client Workbook or can be accessed by searching for this book's title on the Oxford Academic platform, at academic.oup.com.

Introduce Worksheet 11.1: My Current Medical Care to the client and begin by explaining the following:

"We will work together on difficulties that may make it hard to participate in your medical and rehabilitation treatment and may be getting in the way of your recovery. We'll do this by identifying the specific problems or areas of concern. We'll then work together to develop ideas on how to solve them."

Then, as the client works through Worksheet 11.1 with you, try to obtain a general sense of potential barriers, using questions that elicit specific client concerns and perceived obstacles:

"So far, what have you found to be the hardest part of participating in your medical care or rehabilitation? What could potentially get in

the way of doing [X treatment]? What might make it harder for you to pursue this medical treatment or make this change? When thinking about pursuing this goal, what obstacles or challenges do you foresee? What difficulties have you run into so far?"

Once barriers are identified, work with the client to develop structured approaches to ensure adherence to appointments, rehabilitation assignments, and lifestyle and medical recommendations. This will involve collaborative psychoeducation and problem-solving paired with personalized strategies taking into consideration the client's needs and limitations. Depending on the barrier, adherence strategies may require involvement of family members and care partners.

Addressing Barriers to Adherence: Low Motivation or Ambivalence

When faced with an abrupt medical change or sudden disability, it is common for clients to have ambivalence about medical treatments. To troubleshoot low motivation or ambivalence for change, use the prompts and discussion points below. These enable clients to identify and articulate their personal desires for medical treatment and recovery and to express aloud their internal motivations (from Miller & Rollnick, 2012). Provide the client with another copy of Worksheet 1.2: Processing Pros and Cons, and use this motivational enhancement tool to focus on goals around medical and rehabilitation adherence. The worksheet contains prompts to enhance motivation and identify potential obstacles to treatment engagement. Worksheet 1.2 can also help clients reflect on the potential benefits of changing (adhering to a medical recommendation) and the potential costs of not changing (not adhering to a medical recommendation).

"Are there any upsides you can see from taking your medication regularly? If you did make this change, what do you think could be the best result or outcome?"

"Even if it feels unlikely, what could be a potential consequence down the line of not taking care of your heart health? Even if you don't envision this happening to you, what might be some potential consequences for someone who doesn't participate in occupational therapy?"

Exploring the positive consequences of change can also be helpful to the client:

> *"I know there are some barriers to [goal], which we'll talk about shortly. For a moment, let's set those aside and imagine that you were successful in making this change. What might be different in the future? If you were able to fully engage in these treatments, what do you think you could accomplish in terms of your recovery? What if your symptoms were reduced by 20 percent—how do you think this would feel? How could life be different?"*

When asked about medical care, clients may respond by summarizing others' concerns about their health and recovery. For example, "My daughter tells me I should be going to physical therapy, but I don't think I need it." Explore the client's understanding of the concerns of others and why they may have them. This can help the client take on the perspective of their loved one, and process and consider aloud their reasons for change. For example:

> *"Why do you suppose your daughter is worried about this? What do you think she might be noticing? What do you think her goals might be for your recovery? What has your daughter said about your treatment? Why do you suppose she feels this way? What do you think her goals might be in encouraging you to pursue this treatment?"*

Other clients may be unsure or defer to their physician's feedback ("My doctor said it's important" or "My doctor told me to"). Elicit from the client their own thoughts and help them to consider their providers' perspective: *"What do you think about this [symptom or recommendation]? Why do you think your cardiologist might feel this way?"*

Some additional strategies to target ambivalence or low motivation for change include the following:

- **Allow the client to be a source of ideas.** Exploring the client's own ideas for how best to pursue their goals and address potential obstacles can strengthen their sense of self-efficacy. *"What could be a good first step? What could give you some confidence that you can take this first step?"*

- **Leverage past experiences.** Assess acute or challenging medical experiences the client has faced, or any difficult changes they have made for their health in the past (quit smoking, lifestyle change like increasing physical activity). *"Were there other times you faced a sudden illness or other sudden change in your life? What was that like? How did you respond?"* Elicit specifics on how the client made this change. This encourages the client to identify and articulate sources of strength and skillsets that are already present within them.
- **Underscore resources and sources of support.** *"Are there others (family, friends, loved ones) who you could call on for support? In what ways could they be helpful? If you hit a roadblock, how might they be able to help?"*

Addressing Barriers to Adherence: Mood and Anxiety Symptoms

Hopelessness and helplessness are well-known barriers to adherence. Hopelessness can fuel poor expectations of treatment and recovery, and lead to resignation and reduced engagement. Perceived incapacity, pessimism, and unhelpful thoughts can lead clients to amplify their level of disability or devalue the role of treatment. In addition, anxious clients may only see perceived threats associated with treatments or expect catastrophic outcomes. Clients may also have maladaptive beliefs about being considered disabled, perceived indicators of disability (e.g., using a cane or wheelchair), and asking for help (burdening others), which can contribute to nonadherence and serve as an important area of focus in psychotherapy. The severity of these symptoms and associated assumptions about recovery and treatment may vary as the client's disability persists or evolves.

When the client tries to follow up with treatment recommendations, what happens? Do they become overwhelmed or experience doubt, anxiety, or sadness? It can also be helpful to ask the client how they're feeling in the moment, as they're discussing treatment recommendations in the therapeutic session. Do they feel anxious, hopeless, or skeptical? How do they think these feelings might impact their behavior? Look out for unhelpful thoughts such as:

"If I go to these appointments, they're just going to find more wrong with me."

"I'm now a burden to my family and that won't change, no matter what treatment I get."

"I don't see how these treatments will help someone like me; all they do is make me feel worse."

"This post-COVID fatigue has made me useless; there's nothing these treatments can help with."

"I will never fully recover, so I don't see why I should continue treatment."

"I'm just going to get worse; what's the point? I can't undo things or reverse them."

To mitigate the influence of mood symptoms on adherence, select strategies based on the client's specific symptoms, thought patterns, and concerns. Reviewing emotional awareness and self-validation strategies may be helpful (Chapter 3). If unhelpful thoughts appear to be a significant barrier, then Chapter 7 can help to develop a more realistic and balanced perspective about recovery and the impact of treatment. High arousal or emotion dysregulation may benefit from relaxation skills (Chapter 6) or mindfulness (Chapter 5). Avoidance of medical treatment and medical care can also be a target for confronting feared and avoided situations (Chapter 8).

Addressing Barriers to Adherence: Practical Barriers

As illustrated in Case Vignette 11.1, many clients encounter practical concerns, which can have a significant impact on treatment engagement. These include cost of treatment and medication; insurance concerns; transportation difficulties; mobility and access limitations; and lack of familiarity with the healthcare system, such as scheduling visits, registration, and navigating complex online health portals. Ask about specific concerns and the client's experience and level of comfort navigating their medical care. Be sure to avoid any assumptions about the client's background or experience with technology, or their fluency with the medical system.

Case Vignette 11.1

Dennis is a 32-year-old man with an unremarkable medical history aside from childhood asthma. After developing COVID-19, he reports that "I don't even know where to start" when it comes to following up with medical recommendations. The entire process feels unfamiliar and daunting. When he does attend doctor's visits, he feels like he is never on the same page as his provider. He explains that his providers use a lot of jargon, and he has a hard time grasping the recommendations. He doesn't feel comfortable asking questions because he doesn't want to "waste their time."

THERAPIST: *A lot of people can feel overwhelmed navigating the medical system. This is a very common experience, and many people find it easier to manage with some support. Would it be alright if we work together to try to address some of the concerns you raise?*

As the therapist in this case, you might start by getting a sense of the specifics of "not knowing where to start." Is there a specific treatment or specialist that's been recommended? Does the client have concerns about insurance coverage, cost, or transportation? Once these are discussed, use the strategies below to help the client prepare for appointments and maximize information uptake and exchange during visits.

Addressing Barriers to Adherence: Cognitive Difficulties

Problems with attention, memory, and executive functioning can accompany COVID-19 and reduce the client's ability to adequately engage in care and address their treatment needs. Executive dysfunction can make it difficult to organize and keep track of appointments and plan and initiate activities. This can be compounded by attentional problems, which can make it harder to maintain focus on tasks or ignore distractors. In addition, memory weaknesses can lead to problems accessing details of medical recommendations and recalling daily medication or rehabilitation regimens. Clients whose cognitive difficulties contribute to nonadherence may report problems keeping track of appointments, following through on instructions, getting started with recommended activities, or remembering to take medications.

Work collaboratively with the client to identify concrete strategies for cognitive difficulties and to enhance adherence. Listed below are specific strategies to promote adherence. Additional details and approaches can be found in Chapter 9: Managing Cognitive Difficulties and "Brain Fog." Depending on the level of cognitive difficulties, clients may benefit from more direct guidance and support, with additional involvement of care partners.

- **Calendars and notebooks** can be used for appointments, scheduled activities, goals, and step-by-step plans related to sequential or complex tasks (e.g., "at 1 PM call pharmacy to refill prescription for pickup the following day"). Magnetized calendars and notepads that can be placed on the refrigerator can serve as a visual cue and facilitate use.
- **Smartphones and other devices** can be customized to the client's needs and can be used alongside visual cues. When discussing use of these devices, assess the participant's comfort and fluency. Some clients may need help creating a digital calendar or implementing device reminders. Providing assistance to clients in session can help to integrate these strategies and reduce resignation associated with potential difficulties.
- **Basic alarms:** Alarms can be a helpful tool to trigger specific behaviors and can be strategically placed to facilitate action initiation. For instance, place a recurring alarm clock where the medications are kept, which will go off every 5 minutes and require the client to go to the medication cabinet to turn off the alarm. Or place an alarm clock next to exercise equipment or in the room where the client typically performs their physical therapy exercises.
- **Customized written alarms:** Set digital reminders on smartphones or watches with alarms and written prompts. Additional information on the alarm reminder with specific instructions can be included to facilitate action initiation (*"Do my PT, start by taking out my yoga mat"*).
- **Prerecorded voice alarms:** Audio alternatives to written alarms can be prerecorded on smartphones and other devices and customized to cue specific actions (*"It's time to take your afternoon medications. They're stored in the kitchen cabinet"*).
- **Talk-to-text features:** These features can be particularly helpful for clients when they are on the go and don't have quick access to their calendar or notebook (*"Remind me at 1 PM to call Dr. Garcia"*).

Work together with the client to develop a concrete plan including specific steps to manage cognitive barriers. Worksheet 9.2: My Cognitive

Strategy Plan can be used here. Depending on the barrier, your support may be more directive and hands on. For instance, for a client with limited technological fluency, teach them to use their hospital's online medical portal so they can track appointments and view visit summaries. Also, with the client's consent, involve family members, friends, or social services to assist with coordination of care, transportation to visits, and financial support.

Addressing Barriers to Adherence: Misconceptions About COVID-19, Medical Symptoms, or Treatment Recommendations

Misconceptions about medical symptoms and the role and impact of treatment can contribute to nonadherence. Examples of common misconceptions include:

- *"These exercises are too hard. When I do the exercise, I feel worse, never better."*
- *"I'm exhausted when I try to leave the house. I need to store my energy and stay in."*
- *"I've been doing these exercises for a week, and nothing has improved."*
- *"I've never been on this many medications before. It isn't healthy."*
- *"Most of the people I saw in rehab were much worse off than I am. I don't think I need it."*
- *"I don't feel any different when I forget to take this medication, so it's probably not all that important for me to take anyway."*
- *"I've tried diets before, and they've never worked. Why would changing my diet help now?"*

To discuss misconceptions, use the elicit–provide–elicit strategy of information exchange introduced in Chapter 2 (Miller & Rollnick, 2012). The goal is to provide information in a collaborative way, emphasize the client's autonomy, and encourage receptiveness to the information provided. Use open-ended questions, phrased in a nonjudgmental way, to identify and process individual views and assumptions that might interfere with adherence. When providing psychoeducation, emphasize the client's *personal choice* in decisions about their health and future. Explain that your goal is to provide information that may be helpful, which the client can then use to determine the next steps and what's best for them.

First, elicit and examine the client's general knowledge and assumptions about their treatment recommendations. This helps you assess for misconceptions and provide more targeted psychoeducation (so you aren't repeating back to the client what they already know):

- *"Tell me what you know about the downsides of not taking medication regularly."*
- *"What are your thoughts on the relationship between activity and fatigue?"*
- *"Tell me what you already know about physical therapy and how it works."*

In addition, ask the client if there is any specific information they might want or need (*"What aspects of [symptom or treatment] would you like to know more about?"*).

Second, provide psychoeducation and correct misconceptions the client may have by building on the client's existing knowledge. When providing psychoeducation, asking first is a collaborative approach that emphasizes the client's autonomy and can help reduce defensiveness:

- *"I wonder if I might be able to tell you some things I've noticed with other people who were hesitant about rehabilitation, or who felt like their recovery was slow/unsatisfying."*
- *"There's another piece that I noticed we haven't discussed yet. Can we focus on this for a few minutes?"*

It is essential to address misconceptions about each treatment, avoiding jargon and using the client's own language. Explain the role of prescribed treatments in reducing disability and maximizing health outcomes and well-being post-COVID-19. If relevant, emphasize that consistently engaging in rehabilitation regimens is important even when the client feels fatigued and disinclined to do so. Finally, *elicit* the client's understanding of the psychoeducation provided.

Addressing Barriers to Medical Treatment: Dissatisfaction with Treatment

Elicit from the client any sources of dissatisfaction with their medical treatment, services, or providers—both past and present. Has the client had medical interventions in the past related to prior illnesses? What were their experiences? Mood symptoms can lead clients to focus on the negative and overlook or discount potentially positive experiences. Therefore, assess for positive experiences the client may have had in medical treatment. Also, obtain an understanding of sources of dissatisfaction of medical care by loved ones, which may contribute to the client's hesitancy toward the medical system. Dissatisfaction with treatment may also be COVID-specific. Post-acute COVID-19 symptoms are new—but they're also very real. Clients may feel dismissed by physicians who might doubt the severity or origin of their symptoms.

Discuss and process sources of dissatisfaction. Explain that you will work together to develop a plan to address their concerns about treatment. Help the client to focus on areas that can be changed and accept those that cannot be changed. For instance, our understanding of COVID-19 is still evolving, as are the treatments, and some treatments may seem unsatisfying or ineffective. Help the client to accept that the treatment is the most current, given available data. Interventions for potentially modifiable sources of dissatisfaction include helping clients communicate their experience and dissatisfaction in a productive way and, if ineffective, select new providers. If they have specific concerns based on prior medical experiences, encourage clients to disclose this to their current providers. This communication increases their providers' awareness and improves their ability to customize care based on the client's specific circumstances and concerns. If clients are dissatisfied with their current care, provide guidance on how to disclose and communicate their experiences so they feel comfortable doing so (Case Vignette 11.2 provides an example of how to do this). Encourage clients to report and discuss bothersome side effects with rehabilitation or medical specialists, so that the symptoms can be addressed accordingly.

Case Vignette 11.2

THERAPIST: *Tell me about any experiences in your medical treatment that you've found challenging or dissatisfying.*

CLIENT: *I've just started seeing a new cardiologist to help manage some of my post-COVID-19 complications. In the past, I had a provider who didn't listen about a side effect that was really quite awful. I was on a medicine that made me feel drowsy and dizzy throughout the day. The symptoms affected my ability to work and focus, and I didn't have the energy to spend as much time with my kids in the evening. When I tried to raise my concerns, it felt like they were quickly dismissed, as if I had said nothing at all. I was on the medication for nearly 2 years when I got COVID. Even if this medication were the only option, I wish the doctor would have explained the side effects to me; it would've helped me put the symptoms in context and made me feel like I was part of my own medical care. I've sort of developed this belief that I won't be heard even if I speak up.*

THERAPIST: *You did the right thing by raising your concerns. That sounds really difficult and frustrating that your concerns were dismissed in that way. I can imagine why you'd feel that you won't be heard by this new cardiologist. Now that you have a new provider, I wonder if you can use this experience to make sure any concerns you may have with your care or medications will be heard. What would you like to express to your new provider?*

CLIENT: *I'd like her to know that I had this experience in the past, and I want to feel listened to if any symptoms or side effects come up.*

THERAPIST: *That makes sense. Even though you had that difficult experience in the past, these are important points to make sure your new cardiologist is aware of and to communicate to her. This will help you feel more comfortable and ensure that you get the most out of your medical care. How about you take a minute or two and practice here in our session how you would explain this to the cardiologist? Practicing in this way might lead you to feel less anxious in the doctor's office, in a similar way to what we learned in the chapter on Confronting Feared and Avoided Situations.*

CLIENT: *Sure, that makes sense.* [Client pauses and thinks.] *I think I would say something like this: "In the past, I had an internist who kept me on a medication that had several negative side effects that impacted my day-to-day functioning. I mentioned these side effects to my internist, but they kept me on the medication, and never seemed to communicate why or whether there were any possible alternatives. It made me feel like I shouldn't express these concerns, or if I did, there wouldn't be a purpose because it wouldn't change anything. I know this isn't the case for all physicians and that you're a very different provider. Moving forward, what would be the best way for me to communicate with you any side effects I may encounter?"*

THERAPIST: [Give feedback appropriately.] *You may also want to express to your new cardiologist that you find it helpful to know the role your medications play in your health—what the function of each medication is. Therefore, you would appreciate it if the cardiologist and her team could keep you in the loop and provide this background should new medications be recommended. Do you feel like that captures the information you would like her to know?*

CLIENT: *Yes, that sounds like a good plan. I will raise it in my next visit.*

A related barrier may be cultural factors, including mistrust of healthcare systems due to pervasive, systemic racism in the medical system. This is a common barrier that can significantly impact engagement with medical care. Encourage an open discussion that examines your client's beliefs, judgments, and experiences with previous medical care and the medical system more broadly. You can refer to the section on "Cultural Considerations and Adaptations to Treatment" in the Introduction to this Therapist Guide and to Appendix A near the end of this guide for strategies to address or engage with cultural factors that may impact participation in medical treatment.

Preparing for Medical Appointments and Telehealth Visits

For many clients, it can be challenging to prepare for and keep track of information discussed during medical appointments. Planning ahead and using specific tools can help clients make the most out of their appointments and maximize their medical care. Encourage clients to keep a "medical notebook" they should bring to all appointments that can be used to manage medical recommendations and keep track of questions, concerning symptoms, and treatments. In session, you can use Worksheet 11.2: Appointment Preparation Form to outline specific tips and strategies to help clients prepare for telehealth and in-person appointments and maximize participation during the visits.

Preparatory strategies for medical appointments can include helping clients register or log in to their online portal, as needed, and identify required forms to be completed in advance. You can also assess the client's comfort and familiarity with telehealth portals. Practicing using these technological tools, particularly if anxiety or avoidance is present, can be framed as an exposure exercise to confront an avoided situation (or a situation that has the potential to be avoided). As part of preparation, you can help the client identify who they can contact at the hospital or clinic for assistance in accessing the platform.

At-Home Practice

Remind the client that out-of-session practice of the skills is crucial for learning and implementing skills and experiencing a change in their symptoms of anxiety and depression over time. Normalize to the client that the first time they use the Appointment Preparation Form or they ask their doctor more questions, it might feel a bit awkward or anxiety-provoking. However, being proactive will become more comfortable over time. The client should be encouraged to practice using the worksheet for all of their upcoming appointments so they have an opportunity to practice the skill.

Worksheet 11.1
My Current Medical Care

Treatments or medical care you are currently participating in without difficulty:

Treatments or medical care you are having difficulty pursuing or accessing:

Treatments or medical care you have been avoiding or feeling hesitant about:

Lifestyle changes (physical activity, diet, alcohol use, smoking) that you have implemented without difficulty:

Lifestyle changes you have had difficulty implementing:

Worksheet 11.2
Appointment Preparation Form

Fill out this form and bring it with you to each of your medical appointments. This will help you organize what you need to bring, outline your goals for the appointment, highlight any concerns and questions you have for your doctor, and clarify any next steps you need to take.

Appt. Date_____   Appt. Address_____

Appt. Time_____   _____

Purpose of Appointment_____

_____

Is there anything you need to **bring or complete** before your appointment? (Examples include bringing your insurance card or list of medications and completing an online registration or pre-visit paperwork.)

Current Health Concerns

Write any questions you want to talk about with your doctor, or any concerning or distressing symptoms you've noticed or want to discuss.

Symptoms

1._____

2._____

3._____

Questions Since Last Appointment

1._____

2._____

3._____

Doctor's Answers & Recommendations

Next Steps_____ Next Appt. _____

CHAPTER 12

Module 12: Putting it all Together and Managing Uncertainty

Chapter Overview

This chapter focuses on consolidating and maintaining gains acquired in treatment. Continuing to practice these skills can help the client manage ongoing uncertainty, navigate setbacks, and prevent relapse into unhealthy cognitive and behavioral patterns. As the end of treatment nears, you will ask the client to review their progress and set goals for the future. Two worksheets are provided in this chapter—Worksheet 12.1: My CBT Toolbox and Worksheet 12.2: My Contingency Plan (Relapse Prevention).

Number of Sessions

One or two sessions are recommended for this chapter.

Therapeutic Content

Review Progress

As the client transitions into later phases of treatment, it is important that they understand the nature of gains achieved in therapy and their agency in effecting those changes. Reflecting on changes in symptoms over the course of treatment is clinically important for several reasons, and becomes crucial toward termination of psychotherapy, particularly in CBT treatment. First, this reflection enhances clients' insight and awareness of their internal experiences and helps build self-monitoring habits. As we discussed in the Introduction, ideally you should have your client complete brief self-report measures of anxiety and depression (e.g., PHQ-9 and GAD-7) periodically throughout treatment. At the end of treatment, highlighting any changes in these scores over time can increase clients' awareness of changes, which can serve as discussion points for you and your client to identify strategies that precipitated the change, and reinforces the continued use of those strategies. For example, a client may recognize that their anxiety symptoms have decreased after implementing relaxation and mindfulness techniques. This not only helps the client recognize the efficacy of their own actions but also serves to motivate them to continue using those approaches to decrease anxiety.

Reviewing progress is particularly important for clients presenting to this treatment program, as many of their physical symptoms might persist over the course of treatment; as such, it is crucial to highlight changes in emotional and behavioral functioning, everyday function, and quality of life. It is also helpful to reinforce psychoeducational elements provided at the start of treatment surrounding the value of reducing emotional symptoms/maladaptive behaviors in the service of living a fuller life, despite the very real possibility of protracted or longstanding medical illness.

Another way to review progress in treatment is to examine the client's success meeting goals established in therapy. During this collaborative review, provide positive reinforcement for gains made in treatment and explore any internal and/or external barriers that may have hindered the client's progress in meeting specific goals. This discussion can also be a steppingstone for later conversations about areas that need continued work and setting goals for the future.

Consolidate and Maintain Gains

After reviewing the client's progress in treatment, it becomes easier for clients to identify the strategies that were most and least helpful to them. Using Worksheet 12.1: My CBT Toolbox, in session, ask the client to list the skills and techniques that were most valuable in effecting change. Worksheets can be found at the end of this chapter in both the Therapist Guide and Client Workbook or can be accessed by searching for this book's title on the Oxford Academic platform, at academic.oup.com.

Review with the client those therapeutic strategies reported to be unhelpful to determine the nature of difficulties the client had with applying those techniques. This discussion should include troubleshooting difficulties, as needed, which may touch on adapting techniques to be more feasible and appropriate for the client's use (see Case Vignette 12.1). It is also important to remind clients that the acquisition of skills can vary across different therapeutic strategies, and that some skills take longer to learn. Other skills just may not be helpful for certain people, and that is OK too. This discussion is a good opportunity to begin exploring skills the client should continue working on post-treatment.

Case Vignette 12.1

Jose is a Mexican American male who was hospitalized for COVID-19 and experienced multiple health-related complications over the course of his recovery, which resulted in left-sided weaknesses in his upper and lower extremities and ambulation difficulties. Jose began therapy following hospital discharge and has made significant gains in treatment. However, he continued to express difficulty engaging in mindfulness practice without exacerbating his anxiety and distress. In response, his therapist reminded him that some skills take longer to acquire than others and he may benefit from modifying the types of techniques he is using. For example, mindfulness practices that are experiential and focus on external sensory experiences (such as mindful eating, mindful walking, and mindful listening) may be too difficult for him to tolerate at this point, as opposed to mindful meditation, which brings increased awareness to internal experiences. Jose was also advised to continue building his mindfulness skills over time and revisit practices that bring his awareness to internal experiences when he is not in an acutely anxious state. The therapist also recommended alternative strategies to de-escalate heightened anxiety and arousal.

The continuous practice of skills and strategies learned in therapy is vitally important. We recommend emphasizing this point in almost all sessions and reiterating it as you prepare the client for termination in final sessions. Encourage the client to periodically revisit worksheets in the Client Workbook. This can help anchor concepts learned in treatment, and clients can carry these elements into the future. Stress to the client that repeating therapeutic exercises helps them better recall techniques and regenerate habits when they are out of therapy. Additionally, it may be helpful to discuss how using the following habit-forming strategies helps reinforce and maintain newly learned skills:

- **Routine.** Encourage the client to incorporate practicing new habits into their routine. Having a routine improves consistent use and adherence to skills. Examples of this may include practicing mindfulness or relaxation strategies at a specific time each day (morning, lunch hour, before bed), adding entries to Worksheet 7.2: Automatic Thought Record at the same time and place daily, and creating a bedtime routine that includes sleep hygiene techniques provided in therapy. When skills become a part of the client's daily and weekly routine, it increases the client's chances of maintaining them over time.

- **Rewards.** Positive reinforcement is one of the most effective ways to sustain habits and foster motivation to keep moving toward goals. Encourage the client to create concrete benchmarks to meet goals (e.g., practicing relaxation techniques every morning, using the reframing unhelpful thoughts technique three times per week) and treat themselves with small but satisfying rewards (e.g., buy the book they have been wanting, get their hair done, watch a sports game at the venue as opposed to on television).

- **Environment.** The client is likely to benefit from creating and/or modifying their environment to make it easier to sustain gains acquired in treatment. For example, objects in the environment can serve as visual reminders to engage in new habits: Creating a "meditation corner" in the client's home can remind them to practice mindfulness, leaving sneakers and a yoga mat near the door on specific days of the week can remind clients to engage in physical exercise, and taping completed Worksheet 7.1: Common Thinking Traps on the refrigerator will remind the client to reframe unhelpful thoughts.

- **Relationships.** Sharing a common goal with a friend or loved one can keep us accountable and motivated to continue moving toward those goals. It may be helpful to encourage the client to buddy up with a friend or loved one to increase the chances that they will rehearse the use of newly learned skills and self-care strategies.

Sharing a goal with a friend or loved one can increase social accountability.

Setbacks and Relapse Prevention

It is important to make clients aware of the distinction between temporary setbacks and more persistent re-emergence of mood or anxiety symptoms that warrant further treatment. Temporary setbacks are a natural and inevitable part of progress and should be normalized. Inform the client that successful completion of therapy does not preclude them from experiencing difficulties with their symptoms in the future. Quite the contrary: For most people, symptoms and difficulties are likely to wax and wane over time. Advise the client that the best way to maintain treatment gains over time is to be prepared for future adversity. Let them know that periods of difficulty are not indications that treatment was unsuccessful; rather, they are a reminder to apply the skills gained in therapy. Encourage the client to use the resources acquired in therapy to refresh and refamiliarize themselves with techniques that may help them overcome hard times.

More importantly, ask clients to prepare a contingency plan to assist them in the event of a setback that results in persistent re-emergence of symptoms. Use Worksheet 12.2: My Contingency Plan (Relapse Prevention) to develop a contingency plan with the client. Worksheets can be found at the end of this chapter in both the Therapist Guide and Client Workbook or can be accessed by searching for this book's title on the Oxford Academic platform, at academic.oup.com. Figure 12.1 (which appears both in this Therapist Guide and in the Client Workbook) provides an example of a completed contingency plan worksheet.

Make sure to include the following components in the client's contingency plan:

1. **Identify triggering events:** Identify situations and life events that have a high probability of negatively impacting the client's mood. Common examples include life transitions (such as moving, retirement, or the birth of a baby), work stress, grief and loss, health decline, and financial concerns.

Triggering Events	Unhelpful Responses	Skilled Responses
Ex: Being invited to attend social events. I feel awkward having to use a cane around others who have always known me to be athletic and strong. Fear getting into uncomfortable conversations about my recovery and experience with Covid-19. I don't want people to feel sorry for me.	Accept the invitation and then cancel at the last minute. **Short-Term Consequence:** Immediate relief from avoiding the event. **Long-Term Consequence:** Miss out on connecting and spending time with friends and family. Feel more socially isolated.	Practice mindfulness, revisit values and the importance of close relationships. **Short-Term Consequence:** Brief discomfort when seeing and interacting with people I haven't seen in a long time. **Long-Term Consequence:** Get to reconnect with people and enjoy their company. Feel more comfortable being around others and less anxious when speaking about my recovery.

Wise Reminders:

At times you may feel discouraged and question whether using learned techniques will ever make a difference. It will. Keep at it! You've succeeded once, you can do it again.

Figure 12.1.

An Example of a Completed Contingency Plan (Relapse Prevention) Worksheet

2. **Unhelpful/unhealthy responses:** These are the client's previously used "go-to" coping skills when faced with triggering events and/or when becoming overwhelmed by negative emotions. Ideally, these unhelpful strategies diminished over the course of therapy, but the client might still use them in the event of a setback.

3. **Helpful/skilled responses:** These are the newly acquired skills and healthier alternatives the client learned in therapy.

4. **Reflect and move forward ("wise reminders"):** Ask the client what they would like to remind themselves during times of stress and adversity. If they find themselves reverting to old habits, what words of encouragement would they like to impart to inspire their future selves in the event of a setback?

Contingency plans are most helpful if they are easily accessible. Encourage clients to consider storing contingency plans in places they can readily retrieve them (e.g., electronically on their smartphone or on a nightstand).

Booster Sessions

Advise the client that if their contingency plan does not help, they are encouraged to return for booster sessions. Should seeing a therapist for booster sessions be necessary, it is important to remind the client to be compassionate with themselves. Having a setback is not a sign of weakness; it is a natural and common part of human life. Another way to view booster sessions is looking at them as getting a "tune up" for a car, rather than allowing it to break down and require several days of repair.

Managing an Uncertain Future

Fear of the unknown is an experience shared by much of humanity, so learning to sit with uncertainty is one of the most valuable skills to teach your client in therapy. There is likely to be much uncertainty ahead for your clients as they continue to navigate the physical/medical symptoms of COVID-19. If uncertainty related to the client's medical/physical symptoms or the COVID-19 pandemic overall has been causing your client distress, it is important to first acknowledge, validate, and normalize their concerns. Help the client identify specific fears. For example, if a client says, "I fear things will never be the same as they were before I got sick," ask them what *specifically* they fear. This helps shrink large and broad generalities down to size and makes it easier to brainstorm solutions to address specific areas of concern.

Once you have identified areas of specific concern, help the client examine how attempts to control the outcome of uncertain situations and inflexible expectations may restrict them from living a more fulfilling life. Examples of this may include isolating and avoiding social engagements for fear of potentially becoming reinfected with COVID-19; limiting participation in activities that bring pleasure and fulfillment because they are unable to engage in them as they did before; and giving up on a career they have always dreamed of because it has become more challenging to do the work with their medical condition.

Continue to explore these concerns with the client until they begin to recognize that attempts to control and seek certainty in an inevitably uncertain world (1) can restrict their level of engagement in activities that make their life meaningful and fulfilling; (2) can exacerbate distress and suffering; and (3) will be ultimately unfruitful because there is no sure way to guarantee favorable outcomes in life. Gently point out that while there is no way to foresee what the future holds, the client can optimize their success in overcoming adversity by using techniques learned in therapy. If the client is having catastrophic thoughts surrounding their future, use the material in Chapter 7: Reframing Unhelpful Thoughts to help guide the client in developing helpful thoughts that acknowledge uncertainty and motivate adaptive action.

Encourage your client to continue showing up and being present for the things that bring meaning and value to their lives. This is illustrated by Case Vignette 12.2. If the client's condition limits them from fully engaging in the same activities they once enjoyed, return to Chapter 4: Behavioral Activation to explore comparable alternatives and ways to participate to the extent that their condition allows. If the client is engaging in excessive reassurance-seeking and checking, return to Chapter 8: Confronting Feared and Avoided Situations. Remind the client that excessive checking and reassurance-seeking behaviors may provide them with a sense of certainty and relief in the short term, but at the expense of reinforcing intolerance and hypervigilance to threat (i.e., that unpleasant emotions and physical sensations cannot be tolerated in the long term).

Case Vignette 12.2

Jose was an active father of four prior to contracting COVID-19. He would attend every soccer game his children played and would help them refine their skills after school and on weekends. Today, Jose ambulates with the assistance of a cane and has been slowly regaining his strength but remains far from his level of function prior to COVID-19. Jose states in session that he fears he will never return to his former lifestyle. When asked to specify how this would negatively impact him, he states, "I hate being unable to be in my children's lives." Upset that he cannot engage as actively as he once did, he chooses to stay home rather than join his children at soccer games and practice. Jose's refusal to "show up" for matters that are truly important to him, just because things aren't the way they once were, ultimately hurts Jose and potentially his family. In not attending these events and activities with his children, he isolates himself from his family and loses the opportunity to connect with his children in other meaningful ways. Jose considered coaching or cheering his children on from the sidelines instead of practicing soccer drills with his children, which he could no longer do. He initially decided against these adaptations because he felt they would serve as reminders of what he had lost and that he could not tolerate that. Unfortunately, not engaging in such adaptations was likely to worsen his mood even more and take him further away from living a life of fulfillment. This paradox was gently brought to Jose's attention in therapy, and his therapist explored ways he could remain present in his children's lives despite having physical limitations.

Finally, consider using the BRAVE skills below (they also appear in the Client Workbook) to teach steps to build tolerance of uncertainty:

B: Be present. Observe what you are feeling, right now, today, at this very moment.

R: Recognize what you fear happening and the consequences associated with that occurrence. Assess the tradeoffs in your attempts to control outcomes.

A: Accept that you do not have control of how life unfolds.

V: Venture forward in value-driven directions. Use the skills and strategies you acquired in therapy to engage in activities and relationships that are meaningful to you. Ask yourself: Am I moving toward or away from the things I value and that bring fulfillment to my life? Sitting with uncertainty can be uncomfortable, but living a life that precludes you from engaging in what is truly meaningful to you is no better—in fact, in many ways it can be worse. So, ask yourself: Am I willing to face the discomfort of uncertainty in the service of what is meaningful to me?

E: Examine and reflect. Ask yourself how things turned out despite not having 100 percent certainty about the outcome prior to your journey. Were you able to handle the changes and difficulties that came your way? What have you gained from this experience? What does this tell you about your ability to withstand uncertainty?

Setting Goals for the Future

At this point in therapy, you and the client should have:

1. Reviewed overall treatment goals established at the start of therapy (Chapter 1) and identified unmet behavioral goals that need continued work

2. Determined which skills and techniques were most and least helpful to the client
3. Learned ways to consolidate and maintain gains over time
4. Developed a contingency plan to prepare for setbacks and prevent relapse.

As you prepare the client for ending treatment, it is important to acknowledge the client's growth and simultaneously encourage them to keep working toward unmet or newly established behavioral goals following termination. It is worth noting that it is not uncommon for some clients to discover areas of weakness or skill deficits in the process of pursuing and achieving goals in treatment, and these emerging areas of concern should be incorporated into the client's future goals. Refer to Worksheet 1.1: Goal Setting to review with the client how to set effective goals. Case Vignette 12.3 is an example of how this may occur in therapy.

Case Vignette 12.3

While in therapy, Jose identified closeness and support of family as one of his most important values. Prior to experiencing COVID-19-related health complications, Jose reported being a very "hands on" person who would provide support and foster close relationships with family by engaging in physical activities with them. At the start of therapy, Jose's physical limitations deterred him from fully engaging with his family, and this consequently had a negative impact on his relationships with family and overall mood. To circumvent drawbacks stemming from Jose's physical condition, the therapist explored alternative ways for him to connect with loved ones that focused more heavily on emotional and verbal ways of connecting with others as opposed to physical means of interpersonal connection. As Jose continued to work on new skills and approaches, it became evident that he had trouble navigating certain aspects of verbal interpersonal communication (i.e., initiating conversations about meaningful topics, knowing how to appropriately respond to emotionally driven messages, and asserting himself), and this largely stemmed from limited use of these skills in the past. To support Jose's continued pursuit of value-driven goals, the therapist incorporated some skills-based exercises to help strengthen these areas of weakness and encouraged him to continue building these skills over time, even after therapy ended.

Termination of Treatment

Discussion about the decision to terminate treatment should be broached with enough time for clients to prepare. Provide the client ample time to review and learn how to maintain gains acquired in therapy, consider other areas they may want to explore before ending treatment, and address any concerns they may have with terminating therapy. If a client endorses concerns over their inability to maintain gains without the structure and support of therapy, it is important to validate their fears and express confidence in their ability to navigate life's challenges with their newly learned skills. It is also helpful to highlight examples of how the client has already been doing the work on their own and that termination will be the perfect opportunity for them to actualize all they have accomplished in therapy.

Worksheet 12.1
My CBT Toolbox

Instructions for completing this chart:

▪ List the skills and strategies that you learned in treatment.

▪ Indicate when these should be used.

▪ Describe what usually results when you use these skills and strategies.

▪ If a technique was not helpful, are there any modifications you could try to make it more helpful? Do you need to practice more frequently? Or perhaps that technique is just not for you—and that's OK!

Skills and strategies	Rate helpfulness (0–10)	When to use it	Benefits of the skill or strategy. If it wasn't helpful, are there modifications I can make?

To help navigate setbacks and restore gains learned in treatment, we recommend developing a contingency plan. Please read over each section below before completing the following contingency plan table.

1. **Triggering events:** Identify situations and life events that have a high probability of negatively impacting your mood. Common examples include life transitions, work stress, grief and loss, health decline, and financial concerns. List triggering events in the first column of the table.

   Quick Tip: Think back on some of the circumstances that have caused setbacks for you in the past.

2. **Unhelpful/unhealthy responses:** These might have been your previous "go-to" coping skills when faced with triggering events and/or when becoming overwhelmed by negative emotions. Common examples include isolating from others or engaging in negative self-talk. These are the strategies that you may resort to if you experience a setback. In the second column of the table, list all unhelpful/unhealthy responses, in addition to the short- and long-term consequences of them.

3. **Helpful/skilled responses:** These are the newly acquired skills and healthier alternatives you learned in therapy. In the third column of the table, list all helpful/skilled responses, in addition to the short- and long-term consequences of them. Examples might include behavioral activation (activity scheduling), challenging unhelpful thoughts, and mindfulness.

4. **Reflect and move forward ("wise reminders"):** What would you like to remind yourself about during times of stress and adversity? If you find yourself reverting to old habits, what "wise reminders" would you like to provide to your future self? Remember, nobody knows your patterns and experiences more than you. If you find it may be helpful to remind yourself of previous triumphs over obstacles, write them down. If you struggled with learning some of the skills more than others, note this as well. This information provides you with an opportunity to encourage and motivate your future self, based on your present experiences.

Booster Sessions: If a contingency plan does not reduce your difficulties, consider scheduling follow-up "booster" sessions with your therapist. Booster sessions can help you navigate new and/or ongoing difficulties and help preserve skills acquired in treatment. Another way to view booster sessions is to compare them to "tuning up" your car, as opposed to letting it break down and having to keep it in the shop for a few days of repair.

Triggering Events	Unhelpful Responses	Helpful/Skilled Responses
	Short-Term Consequence: Long-Term Consequence:	Short-Term Consequence: Long-Term Consequence:
	Short-Term Consequence: Long-Term Consequence:	Short-Term Consequence: Long-Term Consequence:
	Short-Term Consequence: Long-Term Consequence:	Short-Term Consequence: Long-Term Consequence:
	Short-Term Consequence: Long-Term Consequence:	Short-Term Consequence: Long-Term Consequence:

Wise Reminders:

✓ PART II

Additional Clinical Applications

CHAPTER 13

Loss and Grief

Chapter Overview

In this chapter, we discuss how experiences of loss and subsequent grief impact individuals with COVID-19. Some of these losses may be abrupt and acute; others may occur over time or not be recognized immediately. Grief itself is a normal human response to loss, and you must balance the unfolding and supporting of normal grief processes while also being attentive to indications that other mental health challenges may coexist or develop. This chapter provides direction in how to be present with clients as they identify, share, consider, and cope with their experiences of loss stemming directly or indirectly from COVID-19 and the pandemic. There are no specific exercises or skills to learn per se, but the content in this chapter may be helpful for you to frame your discussions with clients.

Therapeutic Content

Loss and Grief

While loss and grief are often discussed in terms of the death of a loved one, COVID-19 can lead to loss in many forms:

- **Death.** The COVID-19 pandemic has killed millions of people worldwide (World Health Organization [WHO], 2022a). This fact alone is deeply distressing. Furthermore, underlying medical causes (WHO, 2022b), the detection and treatment of which may have been delayed or postponed due to pandemic-related reasons, have been significant causes of mortality during the pandemic (WHO,

2022b). These millions of deaths represent millions more people who experience the loss of a loved one. Clients therefore may present with bereavement related to their personal circle (e.g., partners, family members, friends) as well as bereavement of others in their wider social and professional circles, such as coworkers, teachers, mentors, or other community members.

- **Functioning.** The change in bodily functions resulting from COVID-19 can be experienced as a loss by many clients. Changes in breathing, movement, thinking, and energy may all be experienced as a loss. The client may also experience as a loss their mental health or emotional function prior to contracting COVID-19. For example, a client without a history of depression or anxiety, with a new-onset diagnosis of an anxiety or depressive disorder in the context of COVID-19, may mourn the loss of positive emotions that are clouded or overshadowed by sadness, anxiety, fear, or anger.

- **Socialization.** Social functioning, whether limited by public health actions (e.g., lockdowns, banned gatherings, reduced capacity settings), personal protection measures (e.g., mask-wearing, physical distancing), or individual decisions (e.g., personal risk assessment to not socialize to protect oneself or vulnerable others in one's environment), can be reduced or modified in ways that are experienced as a loss.

- **Religion and spirituality.** Religious and spiritual functioning may change as an aftermath of social disruption, and clients may experience a loss of communal worship, activities, and rituals. This can be particularly poignant for major events and milestones, including death and funeral or memorial rituals.

- **Social roles and identity.** Some clients may have lost employment, either permanently or temporarily. Students may be navigating disruptions in learning with virtual learning settings or hybrid schedules. Recognizing that school and employment for many people also represent key social opportunities, the loss of colleagues, teachers, and support personnel to death, retirement, and resignation means a loss of routine interactions and of future potential connections.

Clients may come to therapy with one specific loss that dominates their concerns or with multiple losses that intersect. Helping clients to cope with their losses, to grieve these, and to come eventually to a place of integrating grief into their life is an important part of your role as therapist. In this chapter—and in the case vignettes—we focus on working with individuals who have lost a loved one.

Discuss Clients' Thoughts and Emotions Specifically Related to Loss

Perhaps one of the greatest challenges for a therapist when helping someone with grief is the impulse to try to make things better, to try to "fix it." If your client is experiencing grief related to the loss of a loved one, try to resist the impulse to jump in. In time, the client will be able to learn and try out new skills, and you can help shape the client's trying of new skills and re-engagement with previous skills and activities. First, though, you must listen carefully, being attentive to the client's story. Stories of loss, particularly of death, can be difficult for the teller and for the listener. Some clients may be very forthcoming; others may not be ready; all will have their own pace. Listen carefully for thoughts and emotions related to the loss and gently probe for further clarification. Your nonjudgmental stance is crucial, as this allows the client to be able to voice their story and bring words to feelings, some of which may seem "taboo" or out of line with what typically is considered "appropriate" grief. For example, this could be anger at the deceased, or survivor guilt. As shown in Case Vignette 13.1, clients may feel responsible in some way for the loved one's death.

Case Vignette 13.1

Jackie is a Black divorced woman employed at an urban hospital. During the first wave of the COVID-19 pandemic, she worked tirelessly to provide sanitary environments for the units under her purview, working extra shifts when staff were unable to work due to illness. Jackie was careful about coming home after shifts, showering, and laundering her clothes that she wore to and from work. She lived with her younger brother, Colin, whom she had helped raise after the death of their parents. Colin and Jackie had always been very close, and Colin moved in with Jackie after her divorce. Colin, employed as a food delivery driver, had lived with diabetes for a number of years. While both Jackie and Colin continued to work during the initial weeks of the pandemic, they both were careful to take precautions such as wearing masks and gloves, and physically distancing as they could. When they both began to have symptoms of COVID-19, they attempted to take care of one another; however, Colin's symptoms worsened, and he was hospitalized. He was intubated but quickly succumbed to the disease, dying without Jackie being able to be physically by his side, as she was still recovering at home. In addition to her sorrow and grief over her "baby brother's" death, Jackie has struggled with considerable guilt and a sense of losing her identity as a sister. She repeatedly has stated, "If only I had gotten him to the hospital sooner" and "I know I brought this home to him—I should have been more careful." Jackie says that she cannot forgive herself for what she sees as her inability to protect her brother from illness and death.

Given that therapists also have personal experience with the pandemic, you may have suffered the loss of someone either personally or professionally. You can self-assess to determine if you are emotionally prepared to work with someone grieving. Attending to your own emotional responses is important in this work. Skills such as self-care and mindfulness practice are recommended. Empathy stemming from your own experience can help inform your response to clients; however, maintaining a connected professional stance is important so that you are responsible for "holding" the story and emotions of the client and not vice versa.

Psychoeducation on Grief and Individual Variation in Grief

Grief reactions can be disorienting to the bereaved person, and you can help by providing psychoeducation on grief. Helping clients to understand their own individual experience in light of what is known about grief can be reassuring. Clients may expect to feel sad and distressed but may not expect to feel angry or detached or to not feel as sad as they expected. Clients may express concern that they are not grieving "the right way" or that others think this of them. Clients may also share they are upset that others do not grieve as they do or do not understand. Providing clients with information on typical grief, and how variable it can be, helps them to make sense of their own thoughts, feelings, and behaviors, as well as those of others. Common emotional responses to grief include shock, numbness, disbelief, sadness, guilt, anger, relief, and gratitude.

Explore How Your Client Is Grieving

Hearing the client's story of the loss, albeit at the client's own pace, allows you to bear witness, to stand with the client in the sorrow that is felt. Listening carefully and inquiring about actions that the client has, or has not, taken since the loss allows you both to assess what has been helpful or not. "Helpful" does not necessarily mean something that makes the client feel better; rather, "helpful" may be a healthy distraction or something that allows the client to perform daily activities. Listening for what the client has shared with others versus what they have kept to themselves can be important. Understanding what the client has stopped doing or struggles to do or has started doing can be useful in understanding current coping. In the context of grief, consider ongoing assessment for concerning behaviors such as increased substance use, self-harm, or suicidal ideation. You can use formal inventories to assess grief such as the Prolonged Grief Scale (Prigerson et al., 2021) or the Revised Grief Experiences Inventory (Lev et al., 1993), or even a self-report questionnaire developed specifically for pandemic-related grief, the Pandemic Grief Scale (Lee & Neimeyer, 2022).

Strategies for Managing Loss

Often there is a sense that the client's world has shattered when a loved one dies. Navigating through life after a death can feel profoundly challenging and unclear. Focusing on the basics of daily life may be all a client can do initially—and even this can be difficult. Thus, continuing one's basic routines can be grounding.

Identifying and engaging in rituals consistent with the client's cultural or religious background and practice, or events that are focused on honoring and memorializing someone, are an important part of healthy grieving. This is particularly important for those grieving a loved one whom they were unable to honor through a funeral or memorial service during the height of the pandemic. Having a special place (e.g., grave, park bench) to go to or creating a physical space (e.g., photograph at home) that is meaningful to remember the deceased is often a way to feel connected to that person. Other examples include being with loved ones and trusted others, talking about the person who has died, and accepting support and assistance with small or large tasks.

Sleeping and eating can be difficult, particularly early in bereavement. Light exercise, healthy eating, and calming the mind and body enough to sleep can be hard but good goals to set. Many of the coping skills and strategies in this therapist guide (e.g., Chapter 10: Fatigue and Sleep) are useful during bereavement. Additional skills that can be used are distraction, muscle relaxation, self-soothing activities, and paced breathing (Chapter 6: Relaxation Skills).

Finding or reinitiating activities that are pleasurable or satisfying (Chapter 4: Behavioral Activation) may feel very much at odds with grief and sorrow but can help give respite from emotional pain and help the bereaved person to begin some integration of grief into life moving forward. You can provide psychoeducation on how "breaks" from the intense feelings of grief can be part of the process itself. Exploring what it means to laugh or take care of oneself or experience a pleasant activity may be necessary for clients who have difficulty with this or who feel resistant to such experiences. As illustrated in Case Vignette 13.2, while you need not push this past the pace of the client, sometimes gentle evaluation of the thoughts a client has regarding such activities can reveal dichotomous thinking or strong assumptions that can be modified or reappraised.

Case Vignette 13.2

Through the introduction and practice of paced breathing in session, Jackie found this tool useful to her when she felt overwhelmed in her grief and with trying to resume work and other daily tasks. However, she struggled to "be good to myself" and engage in pleasant activities beyond necessities. At first, Jackie said, "I just don't feel like doing that stuff," like going to the park as she used to. As more time went on and Jackie still did not resume this activity, the therapist inquired further about what went through Jackie's mind when she thought about going to the park. Jackie shared that she felt it "wasn't right" that she should enjoy herself when Colin was dead and that she felt like she was betraying him. She shared that she worried it would be like she was "moving on without him." With the therapist's help, Jackie evaluated some of these thoughts, including considering what Colin would say to her, what he would want her to do with her life, and how she could move forward in her life gradually, with Colin still very much in her heart.

Sometimes the bereaved individual may need other types of help and additional strategies outside of therapy for COVID-19 sequelae. Resources on bereavement (e.g., websites, books, podcasts) can help normalize grief reactions and provide self-help for coping. Bereavement support groups, whether in person or virtual, offer the opportunity to connect with others who have lost a loved one and provide shared understanding of the experience. Often people find such groups helpful in being able to express their individual story within a community with similar experiences. There are COVID-19-specific grief support groups as well as general grief support groups. Another option is individual bereavement counseling, which can be a few sessions to many and can have a tapered course. Such counseling can be incorporated as part of individual psychotherapy or with a separate provider.

While many who experience the loss of a loved one will in time integrate the loss into their life with the above supports, some individuals experience more challenging difficulties, particularly as time goes on. People who have symptoms of post-traumatic stress disorder and/or major depression should be evaluated for these conditions and treated accordingly. There also is the occurrence of prolonged grief disorder (formerly complicated grief), which is the continuation of acute grief reaction into a chronic course (after 12 months for adults, 6 months for children and adolescents; American Psychiatric Association, 2022).

Review Role of Acceptance in Grief

For those clients who are beyond the acute phase of COVID-19 and are months or years into their post-COVID lives, knowing when to continue to work toward change versus when to accept the state of one's functioning, and finding ways to live with it, is not always clear. You can help clients find those borders of acceptance versus change. Clients may feel defeated by any talk of acceptance and, as shown in Case Vignette 13.3, you can provide psychoeducation on how acceptance can be beneficial and help the client to put energies of change toward other goals that are attainable.

Case Vignette 13.3

In addition to her grief for Colin, Jackie remained challenged by her reduced ability to exercise the way that she had prior to COVID-19. Jackie had always enjoyed the freedom of running, whether outside or on the treadmill, and had been used to going for long runs. However, 2 years after her initial experience with COVID-19, she continued to have difficulty running for very long, even when she tried to build up gradually. One day she was able to run for about 10 minutes and she felt great; however, she felt exhausted for the next few days. Jackie was frustrated that despite her efforts to re-engage in running, she could not do so the way she used to without coughing and feeling demoralized: "I'm just totally different now. I can't get my body to do what it used to do." When a different activity was proposed, like walking rather than running, Jackie bristled, "I'm a runner." At one point, Jackie gave up trying to do any physical exercise because she was unable to run the way she had before. One day in session, Jackie mentioned that a colleague of hers invited her to go walking for 15 minutes on one of their breaks. Jackie said that she was "on the fence" and did not want to feel embarrassed if she could not keep up. She also repeated her frustration at not being able to run. In therapy, Jackie considered the costs and benefits of accepting the invitation versus not accepting it, and decided that she would try walking with her colleague and see how she felt. Jackie returned to session the following week stating that she was able to walk the 15 minutes and enjoyed her colleague's company. She was even thinking about going for a walk along the river over the weekend. Jackie noted that walking was "better than nothing," and although she wished that she could run as before, she was more accepting of how her body moved now.

One key task for you is to inventory the client's strengths and abilities that have not been lost. These may be areas that have existed for the client for a long time prior to COVID-19; these also may be new skills and realizations of strengths not acknowledged previously. Helping clients to attend to these strengths and skills will help to balance the clients' perspectives on their changed situations. Being able to formally acknowledge strengths— whether consistently present, reawakened, or brand-new—provides hope, encouragement, and a counterpoint to the reality of loss.

Movement Toward Integrating Loss into Our Lives

In time, loss can become integrated into the life of the client. When people are thought to be coping well with grief, this is ultimately what takes place. While there are different models of the grief process and what one does to "resolve" grief (Kübler-Ross, 1969; Worden, 1991), these can be interpreted too narrowly, can be unrealistically linear or "stage-like," and can oversimplify individual differences in coping with loss and grief. In recent decades, bereavement researchers have posited a more flexible understanding of processing grief. This "dual process model" involves the back-and-forth experiencing of thoughts, feelings, and behaviors that are loss-oriented with those that are restoration-oriented (Shear, 2010a, 2010b; Stroebe & Schut, 1999). Thus, bereavement work is not done all at once but through an oscillation of confrontation with the loss and respite from focus on the loss. Through this, over time and in one's own way, the loss becomes integrated into the client's life. This means that the intensity of emotional pain lessens and does not dominate, the client can think about the person or loss without wanting to avoid or escape feelings, and the client resumes functioning in life and activities. This does not mean that grief is no longer felt. "Integrated grief" means that grief has found its place in the scheme of the individual's whole life while allowing the individual to be fully engaged in life.

Part of working with clients to support integration of grief is to explore with them how they make sense of the loss. Inquiring about familial, cultural, or spiritual/religious traditions and understandings of death, for the deceased as well as for the client, can help the client to articulate what beliefs are held or where departures from traditions may be challenged or rejected. Helping clients to think through these factors fosters understanding of their experience of grief and makes meaning of what has occurred, including processing the events around the person's death and the nature of the "continuing bond" with the deceased. Continuing bonds acknowledge the attachment and relationship with the deceased and how attachment changes but continues with death (Klass & Walter, 2001). This new relationship with the individual can involve honoring and remembering the loved one and holding and embodying the deceased's legacy. This may include continuing activities that were important to the loved one, acting in memory of the loved one, or living in one's own life the shared values of the deceased.

Special Considerations

The disproportionate impact of COVID-19 on particular communities includes disproportionate loss (Hillis et al, 2021). When working with clients, you can take a broader view of the impact, noting how community loss, unfairness, health inequities, vastly different pandemic experiences (e.g., working in person vs. able to work from home), and inadequate resources all are cause for clients to be angry, hurt, and demoralized. You can validate these responses to systems of oppression and marginalization, acknowledging the reality of their existence, and help clients to feel heard and supported. Potentially, you and the client can explore ways in which community recovery and resilience from the impact and bereavement of COVID-19 can be supported and what role the client may have in this going forward.

Healthcare workers who experienced multiple losses of patients and colleagues are another special group for COVID-19 loss. Even seasoned workers were confronted with high frequency of sudden client deaths; the scale at times was beyond that which anyone had trained for or had previously experienced. Peer bereavement support groups, memorial services, and dedicated spaces (e.g., chapel, memorial tree, wall plaque) all can be ways that healthcare workers honor and remember those they lost during the pandemic.

CHAPTER 14

Caregivers and Families

Chapter Overview

Family members and friends of individuals with persisting sequelae of COVID-19 may find themselves temporarily or permanently involved in caregiving tasks and changed roles. Particularly with provision of practical and direct support, family caregivers can positively impact client adherence to medical treatments (DiMatteo, 2004). However, family caregivers are also at risk for caregiver burden associated with negative health outcomes. Furthermore, family caregivers themselves also may have experienced intensive COVID-19 infection and struggle with their own persisting symptoms. This chapter highlights the importance of supporting family caregivers and involving them in the treatment of your client. Note that in this chapter we use the term "family caregiver" to include family members and nonprofessional important others in the client's environment who provide care.

Therapeutic Content

Caregiving During the Pandemic

The COVID-19 pandemic changed the caregiving landscape. Particularly early in the pandemic (and also in subsequent variant waves), caregivers encountered numerous limitations brought on by the pandemic. These included isolating; physical distancing; concern about infection/re-infection (of the client, the caregiver, other family members); fewer or changed opportunities for healthy physical and social activities and attending/accessing healthcare; and decreased availability of routine care.

Family caregivers reported increases in caregiving tasks, including provision of emotional support to the client, grocery shopping, and communicating with healthcare providers (Irani et al., 2021). With increased tasks came other changes to the caregiving context, such as reduction in caregiving supports (e.g., less availability of both professional and informal caregivers) and more use of technology for connection (Irani et al., 2021). While technology offers crucial ways to connect with others without being physically present—therefore reducing risk of infection—caregivers often are the conduits for clients in setting up and using technology for communication with healthcare providers and others.

COVID-19-Related Caregiving

Caregiver Burden

Caregiver burden is a well-documented phenomenon and can occur within the most loving and supportive of caregiving relationships (Adelman et al., 2014). Depending on how it is measured, caregiver burden is the perceived negative toll caregivers experience over time emotionally, cognitively, physically, socially, and financially. In general, caregiver burden worsens when there is more to do (caregiving task intensity), not enough perceived help, neglect of one's own health, and/or a low sense of social support. Research from the COVID-19 pandemic has documented psychological distress among caregivers (Shirasaki et al., 2022). One study found that caregivers reported significantly greater symptoms of anxiety, depression, and trauma/stress-related disorder regarding COVID-19, substance use, and suicidal ideation when compared to non-caregivers (Czeisler et al., 2020).

Supporting Family Caregivers

Allowing space for family caregivers to describe their caregiving tasks, the amount of time these tasks take, and the ramifications of caregiving to the caregiver is important. As the identified client's therapist, you are in the position of being able to potentially assess and provide resources to the family caregiver, particularly referrals for treatment and support groups specific to mental health and substance use. Furthermore, by hearing from family caregivers about the specific caregiving tasks they are performing, you can better identify where intervention might be useful within caregiving tasks themselves to simultaneously further client treatment outcomes and potentially decrease caregiver burden (see Case Vignette 14.1).

Case Vignette 14.1

Andre has been in physical therapy because of COVID-19. As part of his rehabilitation, Andre has been prescribed exercises and repetitions to be completed at home in between his physical therapy sessions. His partner Sam has voiced concern and frustration that Andre has been forgetting to do his at-home exercises, misplaces the handout of instructions to help guide him through the exercises, and has tended to postpone doing the exercises until the evening and then does not want to engage in the exercises because he is too tired. Sam is worried that Andre will not recover as well or gain back strength and stamina if he does not do these exercises. Sam expresses that he is worried about his own job and the time that he takes off to accompany Andre to physical therapy sessions. While Sam is supportive of Andre and will "do what I need to do" to support him, he is frustrated that Andre is not maximizing the gains he could be making by doing the exercises. Using strategies for participating in medical care contained in Chapter 11, the therapist worked with both Andre and Sam in one of Andre's psychotherapy sessions to identify barriers to Andre engaging in physical therapy exercises. Through this conversation, Sam was able to share with Andre his concerns and Andre was able to convey barriers that he experienced, such as feeling afraid to do the exercises during the day when he had more energy but was alone because Sam was at work. Together, Andre and Sam decided to find a dedicated space in their apartment in which Andre could do the exercises and tape the instructions on the wall. They also decided that Andre would do the more challenging exercises in the morning with Sam before Sam went to work, and then Andre would do the less challenging exercises by himself, during Sam's lunch break, when Sam could be on speakerphone. After instituting this plan, Andre and Sam provided feedback that they both felt better regarding Andre's recovery, Andre's anxiety about exercises, and Sam's frustration in the context of caregiving.

One way to address caregiver burden is to use the CARE framework: **C**aregiver well-being, **A**dvance care planning, **R**espite, and **E**ducation (Holliday et al., 2022). This acronym pulls together the elements that research has shown to be helpful in buffering caregiver burden and provides a starting place for identifying and addressing it:

- Caregiver well-being focuses on understanding how caregivers are accessing their own mental and physical healthcare, identifying what caregiving tasks are not being done, and consulting with social work or other resources. You can ask caregivers about how they are doing and about the caregiving burden via a needs assessment of the client and to what extent the caregiver is helping with those needs.

- Advance care planning, while often done in medical contexts, is still an area that you can prompt inquiry around if tasks such as healthcare proxies and the client's wishes have not been discussed or documented. Sometimes this can be done in session with the client alone and then shared with the family caregiver subsequently, or this can be done in a session all together. Note that such discussion may be a process over time for the client to think through preferences and may take place across a number of sessions.

- Respite is something that the caregiver can prioritize, plan, and pursue. This may involve longer or shorter periods of time. You can incorporate the option of respite and planning for it as part of client goals. For example, normalizing the need for caregiver respite with clients can start to build flexibility and expectation that there may be times when other caregivers can step in to assist so that the primary caregiver can have some time away from caregiving. Sharing this with the primary caregiver in a session and encouraging joint problem-solving and development of a plan for respite can be helpful in such breaks actually being taken and both client and caregiver feeling more at ease with this.

- Education encompasses both information about the client's symptoms and conditions and resources for the family caregiver's own needs, such as caregiver support groups. You can encourage caregivers to ask questions, both in and outside of sessions, and to provide information and resources to caregivers on relevant caregiving supports. By indicating your openness to be a source of information, the caregiver may feel more comfortable sharing needs and asking questions.

Therapy Sessions Including Family Caregiver

While your client with persisting sequelae of COVID-19 is considered the identified client, the presence and involvement of one or more family caregivers in treatment may be indicated, depending on your case conceptualization and the client's family structure and availability. Family caregivers may join sessions on occasion or at particular points in therapy. Finding an appropriate balance based on the identified client's preference is important. Some clients may want their caregiver present for every session, some may not want a caregiver involved at all, and some will welcome the family caregiver to join as needed. When working with clients, introduce the topic of family member involvement in treatment early on as a way of normalizing the approach and maximizing the opportunity for caregiver involvement in the client's treatment.

Often, the family caregiver can provide useful perspective on the client's daily life, changes that are occurring, and information the client may not be sharing or even aware of. Differences of opinion between client and caregiver certainly can occur and be a point of contention both in and outside of session. However, you can facilitate such conversations and, where there is conflict, provide structure and support to both client and caregiver to work toward resolution. If you plan on including a caregiver in treatment, we recommend familiarizing yourself with the literature regarding qualities of client families that can enhance or interfere with client health outcomes. For example, families that support client autonomy and self-determination, are cohesive, and attend to the client's symptoms have better client health outcomes; conversely, those families that respond to client illnesses with criticism, overprotectiveness, overcontrol, or avoidance tend to have poorer outcomes (Rosland et al., 2012).

As illustrated in Case Vignette 14.1 with Andre and Sam, family caregivers are well positioned to help clients implement therapy strategies and to practice skills outside of therapy sessions. Caregivers can be helpful in structuring the home environment and in setting up cueing and reminders for when and how to practice skills, and can be there to provide positive reinforcement when clients practice skills and accomplish goals. Furthermore, caregivers can help identify and mitigate barriers that the client encounters.

Many of the tools and strategies set forth in this treatment program for use with clients with persisting symptoms of COVID-19 are also very helpful tools for family caregivers to use to cope with their own stress. As illustrated in Case Vignette 14.2, by incorporating family caregivers into client sessions and simultaneously providing the psychoeducation, skills practice, and reinforcement of skills, a synergistic impact can result whereby both client and caregiver are learning and benefiting from the therapy. This also has the potential to enhance their personal relationship and movement forward together.

Case Vignette 14.2

Calvin has struggled with breathing difficulties and coughing since having COVID-19. At times, he feels that he cannot get enough breath. He experiences a lot of anxiety, not only when he feels he cannot breathe and starts coughing, but also in many situations in which he anticipates his breathing will become compromised. His anxiety has led him to avoid going out of the home and engaging in activities. Calvin was amenable to the therapist's suggestion of having his wife, JoAnn, join for the second therapy session. JoAnn corroborated the extent to which Calvin's anxiety has disrupted his ability to function, particularly outside of the home. She shared in session her concern for him to have help managing his anxiety; she herself has become more frustrated and anxious about his ability to cope, and she is worried about their future and the impact Calvin's anxiety may have on their three young children. In this same session, the therapist provided psychoeducation on relaxation, as outlined in Chapter 6, and Calvin and JoAnn both engaged in five-finger breathing. In subsequent sessions, Calvin continued to work on skills for managing anxiety. JoAnn rejoined for part of the sixth session and provided feedback that not only had she been supporting Calvin in his relaxation practice, she herself has found the skills to be helpful to her in calming herself, particularly when she starts to feel overwhelmed with caregiving tasks. Calvin then shared that they had taught their children the five-finger breathing relaxation and that he felt good as a father to be able to impart this useful skill to them.

Cultural Considerations When Working with Ethnoculturally Diverse Families

According to the most recent National Alliance of Caregiving survey of caregiving in the United States (National Alliance for Caregiving/ AARP, 2020), people of color providing care to a loved one were more likely than White caregivers to have their loved one reside with them. This survey also found that Black caregivers were less likely to engage in respite services, while Hispanic caregivers reported spending more time caregiving than White caregivers and engaging in more high-intensity caregiving. Thus, cultural responsiveness to families is crucial. Western therapies often are undergirded with assumptions of individual responsibility, while other cultures elevate the family unit and older generations. Sensitivity to these differences will assist you in adjusting therapy and incorporating family members appropriately. Understanding expectations of caregiving roles based on gender or birth order is important. Appreciating too that there may be differences in acceptance of caregiving responsibilities across generations and acculturation levels, you should inquire and assess the family relationships and roles specific to the individual family in session. Conflict or differences of opinion in how caregiving should occur may be based in cultural values, and therapists can help clients and caregivers to navigate these concerns.

Cultural Considerations: Case Vignettes and Worksheets

This appendix contains case vignettes highlighting concepts in cultural considerations as well as two optional worksheets.

- Case Vignette 1 is a brief illustration of how to practice cultural humility while exploring the client's cultural background and perspectives.
- Case Vignette 2 provides an example of how the acculturation process may contribute to your client's psychological symptoms and/or engagement in treatment.
- Case Vignette 3 is an example of working with a client who has internalized harmful beliefs and exploring the damaging implications of these beliefs on their behaviors, values, and goals as it relates to adjusting to the persistent symptoms of COVID-19.
- Case Vignette 4 illustrates how a therapist can explore client beliefs about medications—which often differ by culture—and help the client develop skills to communicate concerns to their physician.

Worksheet A: Cultural Identity Questionnaire and Worksheet B: Cultural Values and Relevant Experiences are provided to help you further assess and explore client cultural identity, values, and beliefs.

Case Vignette 1

THERAPIST: *If it is alright with you, I would like to spend some time getting to know more about your cultural background and perspectives, so we can formulate a treatment plan that is consistent with what is meaningful to you.*

CLIENT: *OK, sure.*

THERAPIST: *I also want to emphasize that we're in this together and will be working as a team. Although I may have a lot of knowledge when it comes to therapy, I will defer to your guidance when it comes to understanding your cultural background and values. You and*

I may have very different life experiences, and because of this, there may be times when I misunderstand and/or overlook aspects of your cultural identity that may be very important to you. Should this happen at any point in therapy, I want you to know that I am completely open to correction and encourage you to bring these concerns to my attention.

CLIENT: *OK, that might be weird, but I'll try my best. That is thoughtful of you to bring up.*

THERAPIST: *Great. You mentioned last week that family is very important to you. Could you tell me more about that?*

CLIENT: *Yes, my parents and siblings are the most important people in my life. My family and I immigrated here from Venezuela and since we knew nobody in America, we had to rely very heavily on one another after moving. We were raised to always put family first. It's what we call* familismo.

THERAPIST: *Sounds like you are very close.*

CLIENT: *Yes, we are. My parents and siblings are the most important people in my life. I look up to them in many ways.*

THERAPIST: *What are some of the things you admire about them?*

CLIENT: *Well, our family is very religious and committed to helping others in the community. And my parents and brothers are very involved in missionary work. I admire how much they prioritize our faith and invest in supporting people in need.*

THERAPIST: *Wow, they are doing very admirable and purposeful work. It also sounds like your faith is very important to you as well.*

CLIENT: *It is, yes.*

THERAPIST: *Thank you for sharing your story with me. I realize I still have so much more to learn about you, and I would like to revisit some of the concerns you brought up during our intake last week. We spoke about difficulties sleeping, feeling sad, and anxious since getting COVID-19. Am I getting that right?*

CLIENT: *Yes, for the past few months after having COVID-19, I have been struggling to fall asleep at night and can't seem to calm my anxiety no matter how hard I try. I also feel sadder and lonelier than I ever did before, and I am not sure why. I know I was anxious at first because I was worried that I would get my family sick and isolated myself from them. But now, I just don't get why I'm still anxious and in a sad mood.*

THERAPIST: *I can see how this would be causing you stress and difficulty sleeping. Let's explore this a bit more. If you don't mind my asking, to what extent, if any, would you say your culture and background impact how you have been feeling or what you have been worrying about?*

CLIENT: *Well, I've been having trouble resuming my usual routine after getting COVID-19. I've been feeling very tired and physically weaker, which has made it difficult for me to keep up with some of the activities we used to do as a family. I also have trouble keeping up with some of the work I used to do as a member of my church. It's hard. I feel like*

> *I am letting down my family and my religious community and worry about what my life will be like if I don't bounce back soon.*
>
> THERAPIST: *I can see why this would be difficult for you; your engagement in family and church activities is very meaningful to you. Thank you for being so honest and open with me. Together we can work on creating a treatment plan that will include ways to honor your faith and family values of familismo, while working on changing some of the negative thoughts you're experiencing about being unable to get back to where you were before COVID. We can also work on developing goals to gradually increase your engagement in activities that are consistent with your values of family and your faith. This should reduce your anxiety, low mood, and sleep difficulties. What are your thoughts about this?*
>
> CLIENT: *That sounds like a great idea. I think that's a great place to start.*

Case Vignette 2

Jenny was born and raised in Thailand before moving to the United States with her family at the age of 9. Consistent with Thai heritage, she reported valuing family cohesion, work/productivity, and spiritual practice (Buddhism). Prior to contracting COVID-19, Jenny worked at the family restaurant, attended nursing school, and taught at the Buddhist temple on the weekends. She reported that since having COVID-19, however, she has been feeling increasingly fatigued, experiences "brain fog," feels anxious and depressed, and struggles to keep up with the demands of her previous schedule. When discussing the possibility of reducing her involvement in the restaurant or temple, her parents became upset and were unable to understand why she was unable to complete her studies within the time she allotted to attend courses. A therapist who identifies with individualistic culture might initially assume that Jenny's issues could stem from poor time management and/or that she should prioritize education at the expense of other valued activities, as most college students in the dominant culture do. Aware of this bias, however, the therapist instead explored how Jenny's increasingly individualistic perspective on attaining a higher education may differ from her parents, create tension in the family, and exacerbate her stress. Through this discussion it was discovered that Jenny was raised in a culture that does not give much credence to mental health conditions, and her family, while superficially supportive of her attending therapy, would often refer to her depression and anxiety as "tiredness" or "laziness," which was hurtful to Jenny. It was also discovered that Jenny's parents did not receive a higher education and were unfamiliar with the demands of a college education, precluding them from understanding the time commitment required to be successful in Jenny's nursing program. The therapist encouraged Jenny to clarify some of the misunderstandings her parents may have with regards to her academic responsibilities and mental health following COVID-19, emphasizing how the current state of her mental health makes it even more challenging for her to meet the multiple responsibilities she once managed before becoming sick. Since Jenny identified with values of both American and Thai culture, she and her therapist brainstormed ways that she could uphold Thai family and spiritual traditions while also fulfilling more individualistic values of a higher education.

Case Vignette 3

Jamar is a 47-year-old Black male who experienced multiple health complications in the context of COVID-19 and has been unable to return to work following hospitalization. Jamar is unable to walk without a cane and is physically weak after being hospitalized for several weeks. He presents to therapy with complaints of anxiety and depression, stating that he fears being unable to return to his baseline functioning and provide for his family. During session, Jamar rejected the idea of communicating his need for assistance with physically demanding activities around the house to his family because he did not want to appear weak to his children. He also shared that he suppresses displaying emotions such as sadness, worry, or fear to his family because it will be construed as a sign of weakness and poor character. Jamar reported these beliefs coincide with his values of being a strong and respected provider for his family. The therapist helped Jamar to examine how his life experiences may have shaped these beliefs and through this discussion discovered that Jamar's beliefs surrounding emotional suppression stem from internalized stereotypes and discrimination he experienced throughout his life. Jamar reported internalizing stereotypes of "lazy, deadbeat fathers in the Black community" and was raised to suppress negative emotions to prevent "giving away his power." The therapist validated Jamar's experiences and later asked him to consider how emotional suppression was an instrument historically used to silence people of color, and continuing to enforce those beliefs could perpetuate the disempowerment of Black men in his family and community. Furthermore, the therapist asked Jamar to consider how emotional suppression may negatively impact members of his family (e.g., Will they learn to advocate for themselves? Will they be assertive to make sure their needs are met?). This helped Jamar redefine his concept of what it means to be a "strong father." The therapist also explored what being a "strong father" means to Jamar and helped him consider alternative ways that he could fulfill this value aside from physically exerting himself (e.g., model traditional family values, adhere to treatment and physical therapy to improve himself despite it being challenging, mentor his children through their own hardships).

Case Vignette 4

THERAPIST: *So how have you been doing with the medications Dr. Sue prescribed?*

CLIENT: *Well, since I have been feeling better, I figured I should stop taking the medications because I don't want to be addicted to pills and have more health problems later.*

THERAPIST: *I am glad you shared this with me. Have you or anyone in your family had concerns with addiction in the past?*

CLIENT: *No, I just heard from people in my family that these medications cause people to get addicted. I just don't want to get sicker over time, you know? I don't want to rely on these medications forever.*

THERAPIST: *That's a reasonable concern—I hear you. We definitely don't want you to get sicker. Have you raised these concerns with your doctor?*

CLIENT: *No. I feel like they are just going to discredit what I say and tell me to keep taking them.*

THERAPIST: *It is possible that they will try to encourage you to keep taking the medication, especially if they see you have been doing so well after taking them consistently. So here is the thing: Some medications can be addictive and cause health problems down the line, whereas others may not. It really depends on the specific medication. However, abruptly discontinuing medication can be very harmful to your health.*

CLIENT: *I feel fine, though.*

THERAPIST: *I am glad you feel fine, but I am concerned that discontinuing your medications may have a negative impact on your health in the long term. Does this sound like something you would be willing to discuss with your doctor?*

CLIENT: *I guess.*

THERAPIST: *I think it's worth sharing your concerns. This way, you can let them know your concerns about addiction, and they can monitor your medications so you don't remain on them too long, and make sure you remain on the ones that would be detrimental if discontinued.*

CLIENT: *OK. But I feel like they are just going to shut me down and not hear me.*

THERAPIST: *Yeah, sometimes speaking with doctors about medication preferences can feel uncomfortable, especially if your concerns run against their recommendations. But we can practice and prepare you for navigating that discussion, right here in session.*

CLIENT: *Really? Isn't that weird?*

THERAPIST: *No, not at all. We can role-play and rehearse how to effectively communicate your healthcare preferences and concerns to your provider. This is a wonderful skill to have and will also help you advocate for yourself when you work with other providers. How does that sound?*

CLIENT: *I'll give it a shot.*

Worksheet A
Cultural Identity Questionnaire

Culture shapes the way we view, navigate, and interact with the world. All of us have unique life experiences and identify with different aspects of our culture. Given the wide variability across cultures, it is helpful to identify and share elements of your culture that are important to you, so your therapist can provide care with these considerations in mind.

Please respond to the following items pertaining to your cultural identity, values, and relevant experiences. Please feel free to skip any questions that do not apply to you and raise any concerns you may have about this questionnaire during your next session.

Age and Generational Influence	
What is your age?	
Please list any historical events and/or crises that may have impacted you throughout your life (e.g., war, sociopolitical movements, natural disasters, economic recession).	
Are your current concerns related to, in any way, your age and/or generation? If so, please share.	
Nationality and Citizenship	
What is your country of origin?	
Are you a citizen of the country in which you currently reside? How does citizenship status impact you?	
If you emigrated from another country, what traditions, beliefs, and cultural practices do you continue to value from your national origin?	

Race and Ethnicity	
Please describe what race and ethnicity you identify with.	
Is your racial and ethnic identity similar to other members of your family, local community, and dominant culture? How does this impact you?	
To what extent, if any, does your racial and ethnic identity impact your view on health and psychological well-being?	
Are there any aspects of your racial and ethnic identity that you would like to honor while in treatment? If so, please share.	
Geographic Region/Environment	
Where do you currently reside? Do you live in a rural, suburban, or urban community?	
What are some of the advantages and/or disadvantages of living in this area?	
Were you raised in an environment similar to the one in which you currently reside? If not, how do they differ?	

Socioeconomic Status	
What socioeconomic class do you identify with? Has this changed over the course of your life? If so, how has that impacted you?	
To what degree, if at all, do socioeconomic matters cause you concern?	

Gender and Sexuality	
What is your gender identity?	
Have you ever questioned your gender and/or has your gender identity evolved over time?	
What is your sexual orientation?	
Have you ever questioned your sexuality and/or has your sexuality evolved over time?	
What reactions have others had toward your gender identity and sexuality, and how has this affected you?	
What gender-related roles, expectations, and norms exist in your culture? And how does this impact you?	

Developmental and/or Acquired Disabilities	
Do you have any history of learning or medical disability? If yes, please list the type and date acquired, and describe how you manage your disability. Do you anticipate this disability interfering with treatment? If so, please share how your therapist may best support you in reducing barriers to treatment.	
Religion and Spirituality	
Do you consider yourself to be religious and/or spiritual? If so, please share which religion and/or spiritual beliefs and practices you follow. Is your faith similar to other members of your family, local community, and dominant culture? To what extent, if any, do your religious and/or spiritual beliefs impact your view on health and psychological well-being? Are there any religious or spiritual principles you would like to honor while in treatment? If so, please share.	

Cultural Values and Preferences	
Which aspects of your cultural identity would you say impact you the most?	
Are there any aspects of your culture that you would like to incorporate into treatment? If so, please share. For example, some clients may want to incorporate religious/spiritual prayers, familial involvement, and/or homeopathic alternatives to medicine into their treatment plan.	

Living Situation and Social Support
Where and with whom do you currently reside?
Do you live with family and/or non-relatives? If so, please describe your household and the nature of your relationship with household members (e.g., close, distant).
Who is your social support system? From whom do you seek support the most?

Health Decisions
Is there anyone in your life who plays an important role in guiding your decisions about mental health? This could be an elder family member, a religious leader, or spouse.
Do you prefer family and/or loved ones to be involved in your care? If so, please describe the degree to which you would like them to be involved in your treatment.

Beliefs About Health and Illness
Please check all that apply. In your culture, mental health is often attributed to: ☐ Fate   ☐ Moral judgment from a higher power/retribution for previous misdeeds   ☐ Misfortune imposed by supernatural forces (e.g., "bad luck," "evil eye")   ☐ Biological/medical conditions and changes   ☐ Character flaw/undesirable personality traits   ☐ Other (please explain):

Healthcare Experiences

Given your past experiences, do you have any concerns when working with healthcare professionals? For example, some individuals may fear being misunderstood, stereotyped, or "judged" by their providers. Identifying and addressing these concerns are an important beginning to building a therapeutic relationship that can best support you.

Overall, do you feel comfortable communicating your health needs and reservations to your provider(s)? If not, please describe below.

Sociopolitical Movements and Laws

Are there any sociopolitical movements and laws that may be impacting you (e.g., Black Lives Matter movement, women's rights, immigration laws, and transgender rights)? If so, please share below.

Discrimination, Harassment, and Trauma

Are there any fears of being mistreated associated with any aspects of your identity? If so, please share.

Challenges/Barriers to Care

Is there anything that may prevent you from receiving treatment? Consider family beliefs, religious beliefs, accessibility issues (work schedule, transportation, etc.).

Is there any stigma associated with mental health concerns?

Have you ever experienced discrimination based on ethnicity, race, gender, or any other identity factors? If so, please describe how it impacted:

-Your self-view:

-The way you interact with individuals who do not identify with similar backgrounds:

Is there anything else that you would like to include in this questionnaire, to improve your therapist's understanding of the circumstances you are experiencing? If so, please share.

References

Adelman, R. D., Tmanova, L. L., Delgado, D., Dion, S., & Lachs, M. S. (2014). Caregiver burden: A clinical review. *JAMA, 311*(10), 1052–1060. https://doi.org/10.1001/jama.2014.304

Alexopoulos, G. S., Sirey, J. A., Banerjee, S., Jackson, D. S., Kiosses, D. N., Pollari, C., Novitch, R. S., Artis, A., & Raue, P. J. (2018). Two interventions for clients with major depression and severe chronic obstructive pulmonary disease: impact on dyspnea-related disability. *American Journal of Geriatric Psychiatry, 26*(2), 162–171.

Alexopoulos, G. S., Wilkins, V. M., Marino, P., Kanellopoulos, D., Reding, M., Sirey, J. A., Raue, P. J., Ghosh, S., O'Dell, M. W., & Kiosses, D. N. (2012). Ecosystem focused therapy in poststroke depression: A preliminary study. *International Journal of Geriatric Psychiatry, 27*(10), 1053–1060.

American Psychiatric Association Work Group on Psychiatric Evaluation. (2016). Guideline V: Assessment of cultural factors. In *The American Psychiatric Association practice guidelines for the psychiatric evaluation of adults* (3rd ed., pp. 27–30). American Psychiatric Association. https://psychiatryonline.org/doi/pdf/10.1176/appi.books.9780890426760

American Psychological Association. (2017). *Multicultural guidelines: An ecological approach to context, identity, and intersectionality, 2017.* http://www.apa.org/about/policy/multicultural-guidelines.aspx

American Psychiatric Association. (2022). *Diagnostic and statistical manual of mental disorders, fifth edition, text revision (DSM-5-TR).* American Psychiatric Association. https://www.psychiatry.org/psychiatrists/practice/dsm

Ameringer, S., Elswick Jr, R. K., Menzies, V., Robins, J. L., Starkweather, A., Walter, J., . . . Jallo, N. (2016). Psychometric evaluation of the PROMIS Fatigue-short form across diverse populations. *Nursing Research, 65*(4), 279.

Balsa, A. I., & McGuire, T. G. (2003). Prejudice, clinical uncertainty and stereotyping as sources of health disparities. *Journal of Health Economics, 22*(1), 89–116.

Barlow, D. H., Farchione, T. J., Sauer-Zavala, S., Latin, H. M., Ellard, K. K., Bullis, J. R., Bentley, K. H., Boettcher, H. T., & Cassiello-Robbins, C. (2017). *Unified protocol for transdiagnostic treatment of emotional disorders: Therapist guide*. Oxford University Press.

Beck, J. S. (2020). *Cognitive behavior therapy: Basics and beyond*. Guilford.

Blevins, C. A., Weathers, F. W., Davis, M. T., Witte, T. K., & Domino, J. L. (2015). The posttraumatic stress disorder checklist for DSM-5 (PCL-5): Development and initial psychometric evaluation. *Journal of Traumatic Stress, 28*(6), 489–498.

Brown, T. L., Vinson, E. S., & Abdullah, T. (2015). Cross-cultural considerations with African American clients: A perspective on psychological assessment. In L. T. Benuto & B. D. Leany (Eds.), *Guide to psychological assessment with African Americans* (pp. 9–18). Springer, New York, NY.

Chambless, D. L., & Gillis, M. M. (1993). Cognitive therapy of anxiety disorders. *Journal of Consulting and Clinical Psychology, 61*(2), 248.

Clement, S., Schauman, O., Graham, T., Maggioni, F., Evans-Lacko, S., Bezborodovs, N., Morgan, C., Rüsch, N. Brown, J. S. L., & Thornicroft, G. (2015). What is the impact of mental health–related stigma on help-seeking? A systematic review of quantitative and qualitative studies. *Psychological Medicine, 45*, 11–27. doi:10.1017/S0033291714000129

Cornwell, B. R., Overstreet, C., Krimsky, M., & Grillon, C. (2013). Passive avoidance is linked to impaired fear extinction in humans. *Learning & Memory, 20*(3), 164–169.

Czeisler, M. E., Lane, R. I., Petrosky, E., Wiley, J. F., Christensen, A., Njai, R., Weaver, M. D., Robbins, R., Facer-Childs, E. R., Barger, L. K., Czeisler, C. A., Howard, M. E., & Rajaratnam, S. M. W. (2020) Mental health, substance use, and suicidal ideation during the COVID-19 pandemic—United States, June 24–30, 2020. *Morbidity and Mortality Weekly Report (MMWR), 69*, 1049–1057. https://doi.org/10.15585/mmwr.mm6932a1

Desrosiers, A., Vine, V., Klemanski, D. H., & Nolen-Hoeksema, S. (2013). Mindfulness and emotion regulation in depression and anxiety: Common and distinct mechanisms of action. *Depression and Anxiety, 30*(7), 654–661.

DiMatteo, M. R. (2004). Social support and patient adherence to medical treatment: A meta-analysis. *Health Psychology, 23*(2), 207–218. https://doi.org/10.1037/0278-6133.23.2.207

Esch, T., Fricchione, G. L., & Stefano, G. B. (2003). The therapeutic use of the relaxation response in stress-related diseases. *Signature, 9*(2), 34.

Fanfan, D., & Stacciarini, J. R. (2020). Social-ecological correlates of acculturative stress among Latina/o and Black Caribbean immigrants in the United States: A scoping review. *International Journal of Intercultural Relations, 79*, 211–226.

Flett, J. A., Hayne, H., Riordan, B. C., Thompson, L. M., & Conner, T. S. (2019). Mobile mindfulness meditation: A randomised controlled trial of the effect of two popular apps on mental health. *Mindfulness, 10*(5), 863–876.

Foa, E. B. (2011). Prolonged exposure therapy: Past, present, and future. *Depression and Anxiety, 28*(12), 1043–1047.

Fung, K., & Lo, T. (2017). An integrative clinical approach to culturally competent psychotherapy. *Journal of Contemporary Psychotherapy, 47*, 65–73. doi:10.1007/s10879-016-9341-8

Gardiner, P., Whelan, J., White, L. F., Filippelli, A. C., Bharmal, N., & Kaptchuk, T. J. (2013). A systematic review of the prevalence of herb usage among racial/ethnic minorities in the United States. *Journal of Immigrant and Minority Health, 15*(4), 817–828.

Gotaas, M. E., Stiles, T. C., Bjørngaard, J. H., Borchgrevink, P. C., & Fors, E. A. (2021). Cognitive behavioral therapy improves physical function and fatigue in mild and moderate chronic fatigue syndrome: A consecutive randomized controlled trial of standard and short interventions. *Frontiers in Psychiatry, 12*, 580924. https://doi.org/10.3389/fpsyt.2021.580924

Gunaratana, B. H. (2011). *Mindfulness in plain English.* Somerville: Wisdom.

Hays, P. A. (2008). *Addressing cultural complexities in practice: Assessment, diagnosis, and therapy* (2nd ed.). American Psychological Association.

Hays, P. A. (2009). Integrating evidence-based practice, cognitive-behavior therapy, and multicultural therapy: Ten steps for culturally competent practice. *Professional Psychology: Research and Practice, 40*(4), 354–360.

Heim, C., Newport, D. J., Mletzko, T., Miller, A. H., & Nemeroff, C. B. (2008). The link between childhood trauma and depression: Insights from HPA axis studies in humans. *Psychoneuroendocrinology, 33*(6), 693–710.

Hillis, S. D., Blenkinsop, B., Villaveces, A., Annor, F. B., Liburd, L., Massetti, G. M., Demissie, Z., Mercy, J. A., Nelson III, C. A., Cluver, L., Flaxman, S., Sherr, L., Donnelly, C. A., Ratmann, O., & Unwin, H. J. T. (2021). COVID-19–associated orphanhood and caregiver death in the United States. *Pediatrics, 148*(6), e2021053760. https://doi.org/10.1542/peds.2021-053760

Hoffman, J. W., Benson, H., Arns, P. A., Stainbrook, G. L., Landsberg, L., Young, J. B., & Gill, A. (1982). Reduced sympathetic nervous system responsivity associated with the relaxation response. *Science, 215*(4529), 190–192.

Holliday, A. M., Quinlan, C. M., & Schwartz, A. W. (2022). The hidden patient: The CARE framework to care for caregivers. *Journal of Family Medicine and Primary Care, 11*(1), 5–9. https://doi.org/10.4103/jfmpc.jfmpc_719_21

Hudson, C. G. (2005). Socioeconomic status and mental illness: Tests of the social causation and selection hypotheses. *American Journal of Orthopsychiatry, 75*(1), 3–18.

Irani, E., Niyomyart, A., & Hickman, R. L., Jr. (2021). Family caregivers' experiences and changes in caregiving tasks during the COVID-19 pandemic. *Clinical Nursing Research, 30*(7), 1088–1097. https://doi.org/10.1177/10547738211014211

Jaywant, A., Bueno-Castellano, C., Oberlin, L. E., Vanderlind, W. M., Wilkins, V. M., Cherestal, S., Boas, S. J., & Kanellopoulos, D. (2022). Psychological interventions on the front lines: A roadmap for the development of a behavioral treatment program to mitigate the mental health burden faced by COVID-19 survivors. *Professional Psychology: Research and Practice, 53*, 80–89. https://doi.org/10.1037/pro0000417

Jaywant, A., Vanderlind, W. M., Alexopoulos, G. S., Fridman, C. B., Perlis, R. H., & Gunning, F. M. (2021a). Frequency and profile of objective cognitive deficits in hospitalized patients recovering from COVID-19. *Neuropsychopharmacology, 46*(13), 2235–2240.

Jaywant, A., Vanderlind, W. M., Boas, S. J., & Dickerman, A. L. (2021b). Behavioral interventions in acute COVID-19 recovery: A new opportunity for integrated care. *General Hospital Psychiatry, 69*, 113.Kabat-Zinn, J. (2003). Mindfulness-based interventions in context: Past, present, and future. *Clinical Psychology: Science and Practice, 10*(2), 144–156.

Kaczkurkin, A. N., & Foa, E. B. (2022). Cognitive-behavioral therapy for anxiety disorders: An update on the empirical evidence. *Dialogues in Clinical Neuroscience, 17*(3), 337–346. doi:10.31887/DCNS.2015.17.3/akaczkurkin

Kas, A., Soret, M., Pyatigoskaya, N., Habert, M. O., Hesters, A., Le Guennec, L., Paccoud, O., Bombois, S., & Delorme, C. (2021). The cerebral network of COVID-19-related encephalopathy: A longitudinal voxel-based 18F-FDG-PET study. *European Journal of Nuclear Medicine and Molecular Imaging, 48*(8), 2543–2557.

Khunti, K., Singh, A. K., Pareek, M., & Hanif, W. (2020). Is ethnicity linked to incidence or outcomes of COVID-19? *BMJ, 369*, m1548. doi:10.1136/bmj.m1548

Klainin-Yobas, P., Oo, W. N., Suzanne Yew, P. Y., & Lau, Y. (2015). Effects of relaxation interventions on depression and anxiety among older adults: A systematic review. *Aging & Mental Health, 19*(12), 1043–1055.

Klass, D., & Walter, T. (2001). Processes of grieving: How bonds are continued. In M. Stroebe, R. Hansson, W. Stroebe, & H. Schut (Eds.), *Handbook of bereavement research: Consequences, coping, and care* (pp. 431–448). American Psychological Association.

Kübler-Ross, E. (1969) *On death and dying.* Macmillan.

Lee, S. A., & Neimeyer, R. A. (2022). Pandemic Grief Scale: A screening tool for dysfunctional grief due to a COVID-19 loss. *Death Studies, 46*(1), 14–24.

Lejuez, C. W., Hopko, D. R., & Hopko, S. D. (2001). A brief behavioral activation treatment for depression: Treatment manual. *Behavior Modification, 25*(2), 255–286.

Lev, E., Munro, B. H., & McCorkle, R. (1993). A shortened version of an instrument measuring bereavement. *International Journal of Nursing Studies, 30*(3), 213–226. https://doi.org/10.1016/0020-7489(93)90032-p

Li, J., Li, X., Jiang, J., Xu, X., Wu, J., Xu, Y., Lin, X., Hall, J., Xu, H., Xu, J., & Xu, X. (2020). The effect of cognitive behavioral therapy on depression, anxiety, and stress in patients with COVID-19: A randomized controlled trial. *Frontiers in Psychiatry, 11*, 580827. https://doi.org/10.3389/fpsyt.2020.580827

Linehan, M. (2014). *DBT skills training manual* (2nd ed.). Guilford.

Liu, S. R., & Modir, S. (2020). The outbreak that was always here: Racial trauma in the context of COVID-19 and implications for mental health providers. *Psychological Trauma: Theory, Research, Practice, and Policy, 12*(5), 439–442.

Liu, Z., Qiao, D., Xu, Y., Zhao, W., Yang, Y., Wen, D., Li, X., Nie, X., Dong, Y., Tang, S., Jiang, Y., Wang, Y., Zhao, J., & Xu, Y. (2021). The efficacy of computerized cognitive behavioral therapy for depressive and anxiety symptoms in patients with COVID-19: Randomized controlled trial. *Journal of Medical Internet Research, 23*(5), e26883. https://doi.org/10.2196/26883

Magesh, S., John, D., Li, W. T., Li, Y., Mattingly-App, A., Jain, S., Chang, E. Y., & Ongkeko, W. M. (2021). Disparities in COVID-19 outcomes by race, ethnicity, and socioeconomic status: A systematic review and meta-analysis. *JAMA Network Open, 4*(11), e2134147–e2134147.

Mani, M., Kavanagh, D. J., Hides, L., & Stoyanov, S. R. (2015). Review and evaluation of mindfulness-based iPhone apps. *JMIR mHealth and uHealth, 3*(3), e4328.

Manzoni, G. M., Pagnini, F., Castelnuovo, G., & Molinari, E. (2008). Relaxation training for anxiety: A ten-year systematic review with meta-analysis. *BMC Psychiatry*, *8*(1), 1–12.

Martins, R. K., & McNeil, D. W. (2009). Review of motivational interviewing in promoting health behaviors. *Clinical Psychology Review*, *29*(4), 283–293.

McKnight-Eily, L. R., Okoro, C. A., Strine, T. W., Verlenden, J., Hollis, N. D., Njai, R., Mitchell, E. W., Board, A., Puddy, R., & Thomas, C. (2021). Racial and ethnic disparities in the prevalence of stress and worry, mental health conditions, and increased substance use among adults during the COVID-19 pandemic—United States, April and May 2020. *Morbidity and Mortality Weekly Report*, *70*(5), 162.

Miller, W. R., & Rollnick, S. (2012). *Motivational interviewing: Helping people change*. Guilford.

Moradi, Y., Mollazadeh, F., Karimi, P., Hosseingholipour, K., & Baghaei, R. (2020). Psychological disturbances of survivors throughout COVID-19 crisis: A qualitative study. *BMC Psychiatry*, *20*(1), 1–8.

National Alliance for Caregiving/AARP. (2020). Caregiving in the U.S. https://www.caregiving.org/wp-content/uploads/2021/01/full-report-caregiving-in-the-united-states-01-21.pdf

National Association of Social Workers. (2015). *Standards and indicators for cultural competence in social work practice*. NASW Press.

Nicolaidis, C., Timmons, V., Thomas, M. J., Waters, A. S., Wahab, S., Mejia, A., & Mitchell, S. R. (2010). "You don't go tell white people nothing": African American women's perspectives on the influence of violence and race on depression and depression care. *American Journal of Public Health*, *100*(8), 1470–1476.

Organista, K. (2006). Cognitive–behavioral therapy with Latinos and Latinas. In P. A. Hays & G. Y. Iwamasa (Eds.), *Culturally responsive cognitive–behavioral therapy: Assessment, practice, and supervision* (pp. 73–96). American Psychological Association.

Palacio, A., Garay, D., Langer, B., Taylor, J., Wood, B. A., & Tamariz, L. (2016). Motivational interviewing improves medication adherence: A systematic review and meta-analysis. *Journal of General Internal Medicine*, *31*(8), 929–940.

Paradis, C. M., Cukor, D., & Friedman, S. (2006). Cognitive–behavioral therapy with Orthodox Jews. In P. A. Hays & G. Y. Iwamasa (Eds.), *Culturally responsive cognitive–behavioral therapy: Assessment, practice, and supervision* (pp. 161–176). American Psychological Association.

Park, N., Oberlin, L., Cherestal, S., Bueno Castellano, C., Dargis, M., Wyka, K. E., Jaywant, A., & Kanellopoulos, D. (2023). Trajectory and outcomes of psychiatric symptoms in first-wave COVID-19 survivors referred for telepsychotherapy. *General Hospital Psychiatry, 81,* 86–88. doi:10.1016/j.genhosppsych.2023.01.010

Patel, N., Steinberg, C., Patel, R., Chomali, C., Doulatani, G., Lindsay, L., & Jaywant, A. (2021). Description and functional outcomes of a novel inter-disciplinary rehabilitation program for hospitalized patients with COVID-19. *American Journal of Physical Medicine & Rehabilitation, 100*(12), 1124.

Pizzagalli, D. A., Holmes, A. J., Dillon, D. G., Goetz, E.L ., Birk, J. L., Bogdan, R., Dougherty, D. D., Iosifescu, D. V., Rauch, S. L., & Fava, M. (2009). Reduced caudate and nucleus accumbens response to rewards in unmedicated individuals with major depressive disorder. *American Journal of Psychiatry, 166*(6), 702–710.

Prigerson, H. G., Boelen, P. A., Xu, J., Smith, K. V., & Maciejewski, P. K. (2021). Validation of the new DSM-5-TR criteria for prolonged grief disorder and the PG-13-Revised (PG-13-R) scale. *World Psychiatry, 20*(1), 96–106. https://doi.org/10.1002/wps.20823

Resick, P. A., Monson, C. M., & Chard, K. M. (2016). *Cognitive processing therapy for PTSD: A comprehensive manual.* Guilford.

Rosland, A. M., Heisler, M., & Piette, J. D. (2012). The impact of family behaviors and communication patterns on chronic illness outcomes: A systematic review. *Journal of Behavioral Medicine, 35*(2), 221–239. https://doi.org/10.1007/s10865-011-9354-4

Saffer, B. Y., Lanting, S. C., Koehle, M. S., Klonsky, E. D., & Iverson, G. L. (2015). Assessing cognitive impairment using PROMIS® applied cognition-abilities scales in a medical outpatient sample. *Psychiatry Research, 226*(1), 169–172.

Safren, S. A., Sprich, S. E., Perlman, C. A., & Otto, M. W. (2017). *Mastering your adult ADHD: A cognitive-behavioral treatment program, therapist guide.* Oxford University Press.

Scott, J. (2001). Cognitive therapy for depression. *British Medical Bulletin, 57*(1), 101–113.

Shear, M. K. (2010a). Complicated grief treatment: The theory, practice and outcomes. *Bereavement Care, 29*(3), 10–14. https://doi.org/10.1080/02682621.2010.522373

Shear, M. K. (2010b). Exploring the role of experiential avoidance from the perspective of attachment theory and the dual process model. *OMEGA, 61*(4), 357–369. https://doi.org/10.2190/OM.61.4.f

Sherman, A. L., & Neimeyer, R. A. (2022) Pandemic Grief Scale: A screening tool for dysfunctional grief due to a COVID-19 loss. *Death Studies, 46*(1), 14–24. https://doi.org/10.1080/07481187.2020.1853885

Shirasaki, K., Hifumi, T., Isokawa, S., Hashiuchi, S., Tanaka, S., Yanagisawa, Y., Takahashi, O., & Otani, N. (2022). Postintensive care syndrome-family associated with COVID-19 infection. *Critical Care Explorations, 4*(7), e0725. https://doi.org/10.1097/CCE.00000 00000000725

Starbuck, J., Loades, M. E., & Chapple, K. (2022). *CBT for chronic fatigue: Therapist manual.* Royal United Hospital, Bath, UK.

Stroebe, M., & Schut, H. (1999). The dual process model of coping with bereavement: Rationale and description. *Death Studies, 23*(3), 197–224. https://doi.org/10.1080/074811899201046

Tadlock-Marlo, R. L. (2011). Making minds matter: Infusing mindfulness into school counseling. *Journal of Creativity in Mental Health, 6*(3), 220–233.

Taylor, B. A., Beatriz-Gambourg, M., Rivera, M., &Laureano, D. (2006). Constructing cultural competence perspectives of family therapists working with Latino families. *American Journal of Family Therapy, 34*, 429–445.

Toglia, J., & Foster, E. R. (2021). *The multicontext approach to cognitive rehabilitation: A metacognitive strategy to optimize functional cognition.* Gatekeeper Press.

Toglia, J. P., Rodger, S. A., & Polatajko, H. J. (2012). Anatomy of cognitive strategies: A therapist's primer for enabling occupational performance. *Canadian Journal of Occupational Therapy, 79*(4), 225–236.

Twamley, E., Noonan, S., Savla, G., Schiehser, D., & Jak, A. (2010). Cognitive symptom management and rehabilitation therapy (CogSMART) for traumatic brain injury. San Diego: University of California. Retrieved from http://www.cogsmart.com/resources

Umaña-Taylor, A. J., Alfaro, E. C., Bámaca, M. Y., & Guimond, A. B. (2009). The central role of familial ethnic socialization in Latino adolescents' cultural orientation. *Journal of Marriage and Family, 71*(1), 46–60.

Vanderlind, W. M., Rabinovitz, B. B., Miao, I. Y., Oberlin, L. E., Bueno-Castellano, C., Fridman, C., Jaywant, A., & Kanellopoulos, D. (2021). A systematic review of neuropsychological and psychiatric sequalae of COVID-19: Implications for treatment. *Current Opinion in Psychiatry, 34*(4), 420.

Worden, J. W. (1991). *Grief counselling and grief therapy: A handbook for the mental health practitioner* (2nd ed.). Springer.

World Health Organization. (2022a). https://covid19.who.int/

World Health Organization. (2022b). https://www.who.int/data/stories/global-excess-deaths-associated-with-covid-19-january-2020-december-2021

Yu, L., Buysse, D. J., Germain, A., Moul, D. E., Stover, A., Dodds, N. E., Johnston, K. L., & Pilkonis, P. A. (2012). Development of short forms from the PROMIS™ sleep disturbance and sleep-related impairment item banks. *Behavioral Sleep Medicine, 1c*(1), 6–24.